The
Whole
Life
Diet

The Whole Life Diet

AN INTEGRATED PROGRAM
OF NUTRITION AND EXERCISE
FOR A LIFESTYLE
OF TOTAL HEALTH

By

Thomas J. Bassler, M.D.
and Robert E. Burger

M. EVANS AND COMPANY, INC.
NEW YORK

Library of Congress Cataloging in Publication Data

Bassler, Thomas J
 The whole life diet.

 Includes bibliographical references.
  1. Nutrition. 2. Diet. 3. Aerobic exercises.
4. Health. I. Burger, Robert E., joint author.
II. Title.
RA784.B345 613.2 79-19375
ISBN 0-87131-305-7

M. Evans and Company, Inc.
216 East 49 Street
New York, New York 10017

Design by Robert Bull

Manufactured in the United States of America

9 8 7 6 5 4 3 2 1

Contents

Authors' Note

This is a collaborative effort of an unusual kind. Both authors have researched and contributed material, and both have done the actual writing. However, the final word on all medical matters naturally rests with Dr. Bassler; and for professional reasons the interviews with other doctors and researchers have been done largely by Robert Burger. Anyone who is familiar with the platform and editorial style of Dr. Bassler will recognize the "I" of the text as his. In the few instances where the authors do not share the same viewpoint the text will make that fact clear.

Introduction

When I first met Dr. Bassler, after years of reading his news-letter of the American Medical Joggers Association, I wasn't surprised to find a man who came directly to the point. "There's no reason," he said without further ado, "why you and I can't live to be a hundred."

Tom Bassler is a scientist who dares to talk street language. Yes, he'll cite the medical studies, and frequently he *writes* the medical studies. But he realizes that the scientific message usually gets lost in translation to the general press. And he realizes that to compete against the modern advertising and public-relations hype, the scientist had better learn strong language or be content to go unnoticed.

—We're constantly told to consult our physicians before un-dertaking any exercise program. Bassler says, "If you plan to remain sedentary, see your doctor first."

—For years industry and government have preached a no-egg, no-butter diet to guard against heart disease. Bassler demolishes this and a dozen other food myths. "Egg pro-tein is so 'perfect' that all other proteins are measured against it," he states. "There are no human or animal studies showing hazards in *whole egg!*"

—Cholesterol is bad for you? "A myth! The higher the *HDL*-cholesterol the better." He adds that cholesterol is vital to the sex life of males, among other things! And *all* marga-rines have the *real* danger: *trans*-fat.

9

—Atherosclerosis is America's number-one killer? Wrong! Old age is. "My goal," he says, "is to make sure that when you die it's because of some rare accident."

The Whole Life Diet developed by Dr. Bassler is not just a theory with general health rules; it's a prescription of a hundred little things you can do immediately to give yourself the body you once had—the body of a teenager. Such as:

Five ways to raise your HDL-cholesterol—one of which is to drink more beer!

Three food types that assure you of all the nutrients you'll ever need—one of which is foods containing the little-known *silicon!*

The knee test to tell whether you're drinking too much.

The crow's-feet test to show how much *smoking* has harmed you.

The most surprising thing of all about the Whole Life Diet is this: though its goal is to let you enjoy a long, full life, it's also *the fastest way to lose unwanted weight! If* that's your goal. For, as Dr. Bassler makes clear, weight is no direct indication of poor health. The plump look may be the healthiest—if not the most fashionable—look *for you.*

Finally, the Whole Life Diet depends on exercise—but not necessarily calisthenics or long-distance running. For most people, simply *walking* may be enough. And, curiously enough, exercise is, as Bassler explains, more a way of *listening* to your body than a way of building up your body. About the time I got to know Tom, he had completed his one hundredth marathon. As a pathologist and deputy medical examiner for the second-largest city in the country, he studied athletes and non-athletes who had died of accidents or "old age" at *all* ages. He established a reputation as the doctor who guaranteed a marathoner would not die of a heart attack. Yet he insists that *everyone* can find an exercise level well within his or her physical capabilities.

The Bassler Rule for the aerobics generation is: Don't act

your age—*walk* your age! And the Bassler Whole Life Diet is designed to allow you to walk sixty miles at the age of sixty, or seventy miles at the age of seventy. What Bassler has done is to establish *communication* between diet and exercise, so that a long walk or run can tell you if you're eating right, and the foods you crave can tell you if you're exercising right. A key guide to whether your cravings are honest messages from your body, or have been short-circuited by modern food technology, is to trust only *whole* foods.

We *are* living in a new generation: the aerobics generation. In researching a previous book, *Jogger's Catalog,* I was struck with one startling fact about every one of the hundreds of runners I interviewed. If they were nonrunners before, they had all lost ten, twenty, even forty pounds within a year of running! Exercise alone couldn't account for it; their bodies were telling them something about food.

This is the only diet that has ever worked, and *continued* to work. It's going to change your life, and give you something to look forward to—yes, even at the age of one hundred.

ROBERT BURGER

ONE

The Secret
of All
Effective Diets

The hardest thing to learn in life, it seems to me, is that the best things are not always achieved by chasing after them. You won't achieve happiness by chasing it! When it comes to diet, the same thing is true. Paradoxical though it may seem, *you won't achieve your ideal weight on a weight-loss diet.* And you won't live to a ripe old age by searching around for magical potions to rejuvenate you.

Quite the contrary: The way to live to a ripe old age, enjoying every minute, is to do the things that bring you to your ideal weight. And the way to achieve that weight is . . . to do the things that will allow you to live to be a hundred!

No, I'm not going around in circles. My point is simple: Correct weight and long life go hand in hand. If you try to achieve one without the other you're only kidding yourself. In this book I hope to show you the common sense of this proposition. I'll give away the "secret" right now: If you diet for a good life, not for weight loss, the weight loss will come naturally. To put it another way: If you let your *body* tell you what it really wants, you'll have a body that can last for a score of years beyond the four score we think is generous. But if you try to force your body to do something it doesn't want to do, you'll wind up in the endless cycle of gaining weight, then dieting to lose it.

DIET MANIA AND THE NUTRITIONAL TIME LAG

Our age has spawned a mania for tricks and schemes and subterfuges to fool our bodies into losing weight. They all go under the name "diets." When *Consumer Guide* rated some eighty popular diets in 1977, they were all described simply as "ways to lose weight." Nutrition was hardly considered in any of them. As a premise, it was assumed that obesity can be a health hazard; almost as an afterthought it was mentioned that certain bizarre diets can have dangerous side effects.

Yes, it is usually desirable to shed unnecessary fat; and it is important not to starve yourself into sickness in the process. But to me "diet" means something far more important than that. Diet is lifelong nutrition. There aren't two types of diet—one for quick weight loss and another for maintenance. There's only one diet! Real weight loss results only from a correct diet that will sustain you over the long run.

Every quick-weight-loss diet contains a germ of truth: the diet results in a calorie deficit. Each day you take in fewer calories in your food than you burn up. That's the only way weight can be lost. And most diets contain some sound nutritional advice. After all, most of these plans come from doctors, medical institutions, astronauts, or policemen.

Then why are there so many of them? Why does one have a brief spate of popularity, then disappear? Why are there diet books on most best-seller lists? And why are there so many weight-loss clinics, pills, plans, and programs wherever you turn?

All of these questions indicate that (1) weight is indeed heavy on people's minds, but (2) quick-weight-loss diets are not the answer. Many of us have lost hundreds of pounds on dozens of diets. The seriously overweight person may need help from a doctor specializing in the problems of obesity—bariatrics. And some of the techniques of the bariatrician may be applicable to the general population.

But I'm concerned here with the man or woman who has no specific medical problem, the person with "middle-age disease": the pound or two added every year after the age of about twenty-five. This is the person who buys books and follows fads "to get in shape for summer" (or the holidays, or the vacation, or whatever). I want to give you, if you're that type of person, a book that will change your life for good, not a book that will give you something to chat about with the people in the office. And soon forget.

Too often the diet mania strikes first at women. The reasons are easy to understand. Women have greater demands placed on them to be slim. Women are biologically more prone to gain weight and more likely to retain it even in a diet-and-exercise program. And women are naturally concerned about food intake because they (still) generally do the family shopping and plan meals for their children. For all of these reasons I want to aim my message especially at women, and perhaps through them and with their support reach the type of man who resists the "diet mania" more out of ignorance than out of lack of vanity.

Lord knows I've had some success trying to bring the message of longevity to an essentially male audience—the doctors and medical associates who belong to the American Medical Joggers Association. As editor of their journal, I've tried to shorten the time it takes for sound scientific conclusions on food and exercise to filter down from the academic community to the man in the street. And our association forms a continuing test group of informed and concerned people, fighting their own "middle-age disease" and in many cases trying to give accurate advice to their patients and colleagues. I've come to believe that the reason why we have a diet mania in this country, in fact, is that there is so much expectation and promise of good nutritional advice, *and so little delivery*, that the average person is ready to grasp at any straw of opinion or "research" to do something about his or her weight problem.

In short, the reason is that there is a communications break-down between the scientific community and the public, a nutritional time lag. Believe it or not, the major health associations and institutions in this country are still working on nutritional information that has been out of date for five, ten, even fifteen years! I will elaborate throughout this book. For now let me cite one obvious and rather critical example.

THE CHOLESTEROL SCARE

The American Heart Association, and a host of other organizations that take their guidelines from the AHA, have propagated a general dietary caution against eggs and milk products. The justification for this recommendation rests on research done prior to 1972—primarily the "Framingham study," started thirty years ago. As reported in the *New England Journal of Medicine*, this analysis of a sizable group of human subjects seemed to establish a correlation between high intakes of cholesterol and heart disease.[1] (Incidentally, throughout this book, I will quote as sources of medical information only journals such as the *NEJM*—those published for the medical community, here and abroad, *without* connection with any profit-making organization.)

This landmark study was readily accepted at the time as clear-cut evidence of the danger of a high-fat diet. Cholesterol itself isn't a fat; it's an alcohol, a combination of fat and protein, or *lipoprotein*. For a time, doctors assumed that cholesterol was involved in the blocking of the arteries—*atherosclerosis*—by the formation of plaques in the lining of the artery walls. They advocated a low-cholesterol diet to prevent this form of heart disease; eggs and milk products, key sources of cholesterol, were to be avoided.

Year by year, however, it has seemed less and less plausible that cholesterol *in food* causes the formation of plaques. First off, it was solidly demonstrated that the body will produce additional cholesterol if there's not enough in the food. The body knows its correct level. Second, it has been known all along that cholesterol is needed for the functioning of our glands, and shouldn't be considered an evil to be avoided. Finally, even where cholesterol levels in the blood seem excessively high (about 300 milligrams per deciliter—well above the normal range of 140–260 mg/dl), researchers have shown that the plaque-forming process may be unrelated to the amount of cholesterol in the blood. And, in any case, other nutrients may adequately protect against the cholesterol/plaque-formation mechanism.

I will refer to all of this evidence in detail later.* For now my point is that *the public has been kept in the dark about the emptiness of the cholesterol scare.* We are still told to avoid butter in favor of margarine, when just the reverse is the right advice! Labels on oils and margarines tell us of the supposed benefits of a low-cholesterol intake. Even such a well-meaning organization as the Center for Science in the Public Interest (CSPI), a Washington-based nonprofit group headed by micro-biologist Michael Jacobson, still publishes a "Nutrition Score-board" in which butter, milk, and eggs—three of our best foods— are *proscribed.*

Why the "coverup"? Vegetable oil and margarine companies obviously have a greater interest in profit than in scientific fact or the public health. The presidents and marketing managers and stockholders of these companies are honorable people; but it is in the nature of the corporation that its employees see their duty in expanding sales and fattening the bottom line.

In the case of government bodies, the nutritional time lag is a matter of red tape. At the highest levels of government, too, there is little in the way of public-spirited action to emulate. Our president and Congress endorse the subsidies of two products, sugar and tobacco, which are demonstrably the chief nutritional evils of the people. (You will see later why I call smoking a nutritional rather than a carcinogenic evil.) This is inexcusable—even if it means jobs and votes.

But there are also excusable reasons for delay in getting the truth about food into the marketplace. Scientific studies need

---

* See Chapter Six. Although I feel the case is clear against those who warn against cholesterol, judge for yourself on the basis of the most recent evidence.

the test of time. We don't know now, and perhaps we never will know, the full story of human nutrition. So we must be slow to make all-encompassing recommendations. For example, we mustn't fall into the trap of assuming that vitamins purchased in a bottle are chemically equal to vitamins occurring in whole foods—simply because we don't know how many vitamins are yet to be discovered in those whole foods!

Yet the nutritional time lag must be shortened or we'll continue to be the victims of bad advice, bad food, and bad cycles of quickie diets.

LOSING WEIGHT WITH THE AEROBICS GENERATION

According to Dr. Timothy Lohman of the University of Illinois, the average American is fourteen pounds overweight. Only a quarter of the population is underweight or right on target. Some are obviously way over; others are only a few pounds overweight. My guess is that, if you took any group of people between twenty-five and fifty-five years old, you'd find the full range of obesity. These are the people that took to the jogging boom with a passion—because it showed them two things about their weight. First, regular aerobic exercise consistently removes pounds for good. Second, such exercise overcomes the damage of past neglect to the cardiovascular system.

The largest manufacturer of men's suits in the country, Hart Schaffner and Marx, reported in late 1978 that for the first time in their history they were marketing an increasing proportion of suits with smaller waists. The same sort of turnaround happened to one of the nation's biggest makers of belts, Hickok. The norm apparently used to be size 36 to 38 inches. Now it is approaching 34 and 32, with an unexpected demand even for 28-inch belts.

Anyone who has been a regular jogger for the last few years has noticed that fellow runners are obviously slimming down. The seeds planted by Dr. Kenneth Cooper with his aerobics charts have sprouted in the running boom.* There's no need to do a survey to see that regular aerobic exercise results in an improved body—both because such exercise burns calories and because such exercise *cries out to the jogger to change his diet.*

Nonetheless, a study done recently for Perrier gave the impression that the smoking and eating habits of "active" people were not substantially different from those of moderately or totally inactive people. Since this report seemed to fly in the face of the obvious evidence, I checked the methodology of the study. It turned out that "active" was defined in such a way that a bowler or a golfer with no other exercise (and certainly no aerobic exercise) could be considered "active." So much for the study.

My point is this: The aerobics generation is telling us something about weight loss that we have never heard before. Never before has there been such a massive experiment in human physiology. Twenty years ago we thought of exercise in terms of calisthenics and muscle tone. We knew that such things didn't burn enough calories to make up for an additional piece of cake or even a cookie. We had no conception of exercise altering the functioning of our glands and thus of our body composition. We thought of athletes as a miniscule fraction of the population, so different from the rest of us in physical capabilities or mental outlook that we could never aspire to their level of activity.

A hundred years from now, historians and social critics will look back on the 1960s and 1970s as revolutionary years. Not in politics or economics as much as in human physiology! If my guess is correct, these will be considered the watershed years— when the tide of heart disease and cancer was finally stemmed, when the life expectancy of American males finally lifted off a plateau established at the beginning of the century, when old-age homes became an anachronism. Today, when an American male

---

* For information on aerobic exercise, you can look at the following books by Dr. Cooper (all published by M. Evans and Company, Inc., New York): *Aerobics* (1968); *The New Aerobics* (1970); *Aerobics for Women,* with Mildred Cooper (1972); and *The Aerobics Way* (1977).

lives to his fortieth birthday, one of his nine brothers of the same age failed to make it. With the advent of women's liberation of the marketplace (and of the smoking room), a similar statistic is overtaking the women. Yet the battle against the stresses of modern city life, I believe, will be won at the dinner table—and in the streets.

The joggers who are seen daily circling their blocks or heading to the track have changed far more than suit sizes and belt measurements. Life insurance companies used to have several categories in which to classify their customers. Their actuarial tables were based on those models. Recently they've had to revise their categories to include a growing "athlete" group.

DIET AND THE NEW MEDICINE

In a later chapter we will see also how the field of preventive medicine has been irrevocably changed by the impact of aerobics. Call it "holistic," or "orthomolecular," or "biomedical," or even "wellness" medicine—the role of cardiovascular exercise in this trend is unmistakable.

And if you want to lose weight nowadays you must also take into account a different trend, parallel and equally revolutionary. This is the field of vitamin and mineral therapy—the key to much of the "wellness" medicine referred to above.

Most of us are simply not aware that vitamin research is still in its infancy. Pioneers like Linus Pauling have had to bear the brunt of scoffing from medical authorities. "Megavitamin therapy" is often pictured as the quackery of cultists. And it's true, as nutritionist George Briggs of the University of California says, that 95 percent of the medical fraternity sees no need for vitamin supplementation if the Recommended Daily Allowances are met by the diet. Or even if they're not. As we shall see, the very infancy of the field is the reason why we should pay great attention to recent discoveries, and not allow the few gross things we know about vitamins and minerals to become ossified into monuments.

Indeed, my plea to you in general is to approach your nutritional needs with a completely open mind. Don't allow the discoveries and formulations of the recent past to become absolute laws. Don't be like the generals who are always fighting the previous war. I don't have to repeat the well-documented fact that nutrition is seldom a specialty or even an interest of a medical doctor. As in the past, you're going to have to look for up-to-date advice on eating from the Adele Davises of the world. You're going to have to run the risk of being considered a health nut or a food faddist. But, as the CSPI editorialized in 1975:

> Food faddism is indeed a serious problem. But we have to recognize that the guru of food faddism is not Adelle Davis, but Betty Crocker. The true food faddists are not those who eat raw broccoli, wheat germ, and yogurt, but those who start the day on Breakfast Squares, gulp down bottle after bottle of soda pop, and snack on candy and Twinkies.[2]

Today we are all bombarded with contradictory rules and tips about nutrition. Some of the best-meaning critics of junk food still warn us against butter and eggs. Others see a conspiracy in additives such as BHT and nitrates (on balance, as we shall see, they're OK). The excellent "Nutrition Scoreboard" rates potato chips, which contain more sugar than salt and sometimes no potatoes at all, above popcorn; the eminent Dr. Carl C. Pfeiffer, director of the Brain Bio Center at Princeton, recommends popcorn as one of the few cereals you can bring unadulterated into your home. Should we switch to skim milk, or back to whole milk? Should we eat more polyunsaturated fats, such as those in margarine? As early as 1974, extensive studies at the University of Illinois showed that the worst danger of atherosclerosis is from the *trans*-fat in margarine.

In my presentation of the Whole Life Diet, I will rely heavily on such reports, and I will cite my sources—not so much to aid you in further reading or research of your own as to be clear about what my opinions are and what is demonstrated fact. I will return again and again to the "secret" of all effective diets: You must learn to listen to your body, to your cravings, to your natural impulses.

What if you crave chocolates and Big Macs and Twinkies? The message from your body has been garbled. The two major garblers in our era are sugar and salt. As Richard de Rochemont says in *Eating in America,* our taste buds are "infinitely less varied than they used to be" because of the leveling effect of the widespread use of sugar and salt in processed foods. Dr. Abram Hoffer, a nutritional researcher I will refer to often, puts the matter this way:

> Your palate is an effective mechanism for determining your optimum needs. The appetite-regulating mechanism in the brain . . . and the taste buds combine to tell your palate what you need and want, provided it is not perverted by a nutrient alteration or deficiency in food. High-protein foods are generally more palatable, and most people will consume enough if they **are** available. Yet, you can fool your palate with corrupters—sugar and salt—and most people use them to excess.[3]

With this preamble, I will now go to the specifics of how to read the messages from your body, and how to do the things that will make the message loud and clear.

TWO

How to Lose Weight and Gain Health

You're probably reading this book because you want to lose weight. That's likely to be a good idea; more Americans are overweight than not. But losing weight may not be good for *you*, and if you lose weight *without gaining health*, it's as hazardous as being too heavy.

If you're serious about your desire to lose weight and gain health, there are some questions you should ask before you start. By the end of this chapter, you'll be able to answer them yourself:

1. What's dangerous about obesity—why are *most* fat people in worse health than thin people? Why are some fat people quite healthy?
2. How much weight loss is a *true* loss? When you lose weight, what determines whether it comes right back or stays off?
3. Why do some people stay slender while others add a few pounds each year?
4. Is willpower important when cutting calories?

5. Why is weight loss sometimes dangerous? What caused the sudden deaths in patients on the liquid protein diets?
6. How do you know whether you are becoming healthier as the pounds melt away?

Such questions should come to you when you think of tampering with your lifestyle. There is always room for improvement, but there is also room for error. *Instinct* is probably your most valuable tool. You probably already know, instinctively, what is good for you; but for reasons of expediency, your health is slipping away. You find it expedient to ride instead of walk. School buses, elevators, and automobiles have robbed you of needed daily exercise. Fast foods are expedient, but they have all "vital nutrients" processed out, robbing you again! Economics robs you, too: wheeled traffic is economically more vital to the city than pedestrian, so you can't walk a mile in any direction without stopping several times to wait for the trucks and cars to pass. Calories must be stable to be economically profitable to the city. Therefore the food industry must deal in packages that have a long shelf life—and we find most of our "vitamins" are artificially added chemicals.

The city can't worry about your exercise and diet; so *you* have to worry about it. You must *think* about your own lifestyle; no one else will do it for you!

PROCESSED FOODS AND THE CRAVING FOR WHAT'S NOT THERE

Most fat people got that way because "hunger" or "cravings for food" forced them to eat more calories than they needed. Evolution equipped us with strong cravings that are very useful for survival. But modern cities have tricked us in several ways that make us fat. When we eat a certain food to satisfy a craving, we may be getting nothing but fattening empty calories; the nutrient we were searching for has been removed by processing and cooking. A common example is iron.

Many adults are walking around with low body-stores of iron. *Their bodies keep telling them* to eat and eat, in an attempt to get the needed iron. Bread is made from flour that has had its bran removed—and with the bran goes the iron. But, you say, the flour was "enriched" with added iron. Maybe. Some iron compounds are usable by your body, or "biologically available"; others are not. Your body waits until it has enough *useful* iron before telling you to stop eating. The extra bread you must eat can make you fat while you still don't have enough useful iron!

But so many things include added iron these days that it is hard to imagine how anyone can be low in iron. Some people, in fact, get too much iron, while missing other vital nutrients. There are many other nutrients—some are metals like zinc and copper; others are complex molecules like the amino acids and vitamins. Iron is just an index of the nutrients that are in unprocessed foods. No chemist is going to succeed in duplicating *food!* So the way to get all the nutrients is to avoid processed foods as much as possible. Only by eating things that are *alive* can you hope to duplicate the nutrients that you need to stay alive and healthy.

Lack of a single amino acid makes it difficult to process protein; *so your body should signal you* to keep eating until the deficiency of that amino acid is corrected. Lack of zinc should signal you to keep eating too. Thus, you could well be overweight and still be deficient in several nutrients if you ate "empty calories" to satisfy your important *natural cravings.* If the foods are 20 percent low in nutrients, you have to eat 20 percent more calories to satisfy your "hunger," and you continue to gain weight. Cutting back 20 percent would not be healthy, because it would leave you deficient!

So we see that "the disease of obesity" is more than just extra fat on the body; it is a variety of deficiencies that trigger excessive eating. Low levels of iron cause anemia, of course; and low levels of an amino acid result in "poor protein." But the results of a processed diet can go much further than meets the eye. Low levels of silicon, as we will see, actually result in accelerated aging. Thus we observe that most fat people suffer the "diseases of old age" earlier than thin people. However, I must stress again that it is the *deficiency* of a nutrient, probably silicon, that accelerates the aging process, not just the extra fat itself.

By the same token, fat people can be healthy if they are not deficient in anything! Your great-grandmother may have produced a huge array of tempting dishes at every meal and fattened up all your relatives of that era—but kept them healthy at the same time. They were fat and healthy, keeping their extra stored fat for "lean years" that never came. Many vigorous oldsters who live beyond their tenth decade have had periods of obesity without apparent ill effects. They work hard, play hard, and have an active sex life, while their descendants, with the same genes, end up in the hospital or the cemetery long before that age. Obesity is *usually* a disease, but not always. If you eat the right foods, avoid tobacco, and remain active, you can put on weight without being diseased. But if your diet lacks nutrients, *or* if you smoke, *or* if you remain inactive, then obesity *can* cause disease!

THE FIRST KEY NUTRIENT: SILICON

Food in the city is quiet, the *crunch* is gone—and along with the crunch, the nutrients are gone. The need to crunch on hard, noisy food is probably genetically determined, dating back to our remote ancestors. Exploring a new environment exposed early primates to a variety of unfamiliar seeds and roots—items not used for food before. Body fat could supply energy for the lean months; however, a *daily need to crunch*—to grind with molars on dry, brittle things—forced our ancestors to chew on almost anything they could get into their mouths. This was valuable, for it forced the discovery of edible roots, nuts, and seeds. (Dangerous items were quickly identified by their effects on the pioneer taste-bud scientists.) The noisy crunching proved soothing to the nerves—like chanting your mantra—and so provided its own reward, not necessarily related to caloric intake. You and I also need this "daily crunch."

All that crunches is not soothing, however. Celery, lettuce, apples, and other watery items sound noisy when you eat them, but they do not satisfy this "need to crunch." Odd as it may sound, they do not produce the proper types of noise when eaten. They do not satisfy and soothe you, so you continue to eat. The proper sound is produced by dry seeds, nuts, and cereals—a solid, brittle crunch that vibrates the skull bones, soothing the brain stem, and relaxing you so you can *stop* your eating, *stop* taking on calories!

The proper crunch signifies the presence of an element in food that you hear little about. Yet it's the most common mineral of all: *silicon.* The "need to crunch" led us to high-fiber foods—cereal grains with bran (hulls) being the most important today. Cereal bran brings with it a variety of important nutrients, among them silicon (the same element that sand is made of). Silicon is used by animals and plants to make hard structures—skeletons and armor—and the collagen in bone and tendon, hair, nails, hooves, grain hulls, fruit pectin, and the like. Silicon takes part in the biochemistry of life by making structures stronger; the silicon molecule forms cross-links between hydrocarbon chains and increases the stability of the tissue.

Modern food has the bran and other silicon-rich plant skeletons processed out, making the food soft, crunchless—and a poor source of this vital nutrient, silicon. Human-autopsy studies show that the amount of arthritis and atherosclerosis is inversely proportional to the tissue levels of silicon. What this means is that those who eat a low-fiber diet suffer more heart attack, stroke, and arthritis *because* they eat food that has no crunch!

Therefore, searching for more crunch is important. If we eat crunchy food we will be satisfied more easily—eating fewer calories and remaining thin. Also, the crunchy foods offer another nice property of silicon: They protect us from many diseases. This is one reason why thin people are healthier—they have more silicon in their noisy, satisfying diet! Fat people are fat because they must eat more of their quiet foods to get their "daily crunch," and they end up deficient in silicon! As we will see, silicon-rich foods are one of the three food types on which the Whole Life Diet is based.

The food processors have produced dry foods with *artificial crunch* that satisfy your need for crunch without giving you silicon and the other nutrients. This fools you into being satisfied while being deficient; thus you can remain thin but still be unhealthy, and so have arthritis, heart attack, and stroke. Remember, the crunch of processed foods does not count! It is soothing, but it doesn't satisfy your body's needs for vital nutrients.

THE SECOND KEY NUTRIENT: FRIENDLY FAT

There are *friendly* fats that are biologically good for you, and there are *unfriendly* fats that can kill you. A pound of fat is not simply an extra pound of body weight. It could be good energy, ready for any emergency; or it could be dangerous oils slowly aging your entire body, draining vital energy, and making you ugly at the same time!

The friendly fats are, by definition, biologically useful. All cells in our bodies contain important fat molecules—cell walls are membranes made up of layers of protein and fat. The fat is useful in keeping watery fluids where they belong. Fat supplies us with important hormones, like the sex hormones and cholesterol-based steroids like cortisone. Large amounts of fat are used in the brain, rather like insulation around the electric wiring in our house. Fat is everywhere, and it is good.

Many forms of life also use fat to store energy. Living things that hibernate use stored fat for fuel while they sleep. We have heard of bears sleeping through winter in caves, using stored fat for energy. Seeds and nuts do the same thing: wheat-germ oil is the fuel for the cereal grain to "sleep" through the winter and then spring to life, producing a green plant when the weather gets warmer. Eggs from all life forms are high in fat, because this is a good way to pack a lot of biological energy into a small space. The hen lays an egg that becomes a chick. The efficiency is amazing; the chick is very close to the egg in size and weight! Thus an egg must be a very good source of all the vital nutrients we need for life. Cereal grains, whole and raw, must also be a safe source of all nutrients, including fat.

A friendly fat is fat high in *essential fatty acids* (EFAs)—

nutrients that are essential for humans. Foods high in EFAs are the grains, seeds, nuts, and eggs—things designed by nature to "sleep" for a while and then produce a whole living thing like a plant or a chick. If we eat a diet high in EFAs, then our body fat will be high in EFAs. We will have "friendly fat"—and can be obese and healthy at the same time. Human-autopsy studies show that death from heart attack and stroke is rare in cases where body fat is high in EFAs! Unfortunately, cooking and processing food destroy EFAs, along with their vitamin E. (This vitamin E is crucial—as we will see.)

The unfriendly fats are, by definition, low in EFA. They have their EFAs destroyed or removed. To understand how this happens, you must visualize the EFA as a delicate molecule with a chain of carbon atoms. The carbon atom (represented by the chemical symbol C) is held to other atoms by *bonds* like this:

$$-C-C-C-C-C-$$

That chain shows only two bonds for each atom—one to the left and one to the right. (For simplicity, we'll ignore what happens at the ends of the chains.) A carbon atom can make four bonds, though. Two bonds are with the adjoining carbon atoms; the other two bonds, off to the sides of the main chain, often connect to hydrogen atoms (H):

$$\begin{array}{cccccc}
H & H & H & H & H \\
| & | & | & | & | \\
-C-&C-&C-&C-&C-&C- \\
| & | & | & | & | \\
H & H & H & H & H
\end{array}$$

If all four bonds are taken up with hydrogen that way, the chain is *saturated*. The chain is called a *hydrocarbon chain*— very strong, and the basis for biological life. It is so strong that it can be used for fuel only with a lot of work—work done by *enzymes*.

But for some biological activity, speed is needed. Thus we find that the EFAs are not fully saturated. They have "open" double bonds for biological activity. The double bonds ($C=C$ in the diagram below) are chemically active because they lack two hydrogen atoms; that means they can react with other atoms or molecules that come by. When there is more than one set of open bonds, the molecule is *polyunsaturated,* and the chain looks like this:

$$\begin{array}{ccccccccc} H & H & H & H & H & H & H & H & H \\ | & | & | & | & | & | & | & | & | \\ -C & -C & -C & = C & -C & -C & = C & -C & -C- \\ | & | & & | & | & & | & | & | \\ H & H & & & H & & & H & H \end{array}$$

Because they are so ready to react with other atoms, polyunsaturated fats are easily destroyed by adding oxygen. Any polyunsaturated oil will oxidize—turn rancid—given enough time, heat, and air. Cooking is bad for EFAs. Time is bad also. Last year's crop of seeds and grain will not be as high in EFAs as this year's crop. If you kill the seed, it immediately starts to lose EFAs. Old whole-wheat flour will taste rancid if you chew a bit of it raw.

THE THIRD KEY NUTRIENT: ANTIOXIDANTS

However, if the wheat is left intact, alive, it can survive the winter. There is a built-in *antioxidant,* vitamin E, that protects EFAs from oxidation. This vitamin E also protects EFAs in your body. So it is not surprising that there are theories that taking extra vitamin E might be good for you. Foods containing antioxidants such as vitamins E and C are the third key to the Whole Life Diet. If you take in enough of them in your diet, you'll be protecting the EFAs, keeping them from turning from friendly fats to unfriendly fats.

Later we'll discuss *how* to get adequate supplies of antioxidants; right now, let's see what happens if we don't.

HYDROGENATION AND *TRANS*-FATS

Oils, as we saw, turn rancid when they oxidize. Unfortunately, industry has found a way to prevent edible oils from becoming rancid. Hydrogen is added to the polyunsaturates to fill up the open double bonds—thus saturating them. Look for the word "hydrogenated" on the label. This results in a hardened fat that has a long shelf life and a pleasant taste. Good for retailers, bad for you! All margarines are solid at room temperature and therefore must contain hydrogenated oils. Almost all vegetable shortenings contain such things as hydrogenated soy oil.

These hydrogenated oils are very low in EFA, because during the industrial process of making the oils hard, there are other changes in the molecules that are biologically unfavorable. Some of the polyunsaturated molecules rotate and change into shapes that do not appear in natural foods. These changed fats are called *trans*-fat (a chemical term for fats that are changed, transformed into new and unnatural chemical structures). They can be used in animal studies to produce atherosclerosis quite easily; it must be assumed they are dangerous for humans too. To the extent that margarines contain hydrogenated oil, they have dangerously high levels of *trans*-fat. Most processed food contains some hydrogenated vegetable oils, because they are stable and add to the shelf life. They taste pretty good, so our natural biological cravings can be fooled. Our bodies accept the *trans*-fat, but can't do anything with it but store it—causing high levels of *trans*-fat in tissues. This type of body fat would have to be considered very unfriendly!

Lard and tallow are animal fats from pork and beef. They are natural forms of saturated fat. When humans make body fat from other excess calories, a saturated fat is made. Since saturated fat lacks double bonds, it is low in EFAs, of course. But lard is not nearly as dangerous as the artificially hydrogenated *trans*-fat. A good lesson in the nutritional value of fats can be learned from the animal-feeding experiments using a variety of fats.

Pigs were used in one of these studies. They were put on a 40 percent fat diet, but a variety of fats were used. After a while, the pigs were autopsied, and atherosclerosis was searched for.

The 40 percent level of fat means that 40 percent of the pig's calories came from fats or oils—about the same as the average American diet. Atherosclerosis looks the same in the pigs as it does in humans—blood vessels narrowed by fatty thickenings containing lots of cholesterol and very little EFA.

The fats used were similar to things in our diet: butter, margarine, eggs, beef tallow, etc.

The pig autopsies made a lot of sense! The most severe disease was caused by the *trans*-fat, margarines, and other hydrogenated vegetable oils. The important thing about *trans*-fat is that it is so toxic that it produced atherosclerosis when the EFA levels were normal. In other words, adequate EFA intake did not protect against *trans*-fat! Think about that. EFAs *can* protect you against the naturally saturated fats like eggs, butter, lard, and tallow, but they cannot protect against *trans*-fat in hydrogenated vegetable oil.

(Experiments on monkeys also showed the rapid production of atherosclerosis using hydrogenated vegetable oils. Peanut oil was hydrogenated and fed to monkeys for only five months. Autopsies showed atherosclerosis in this short time. When you count the numbers of "hard" peanut-butter sandwiches eaten by children, you can see why teenagers can develop atherosclerosis! * The monkey studies went on to show reversal of the disease using the same amount of vegetable oil in the liquid form. Both diets had 40 percent of their calories from fat, but one caused atherosclerosis and one removed it. The healthy diet that removed the disease was very high in EFAs.)

The pigs that were fed grease—or "used fat"—had less disease than those fed *trans*-fat. Grease comes from fried foods, especially from deep-fried fast foods. Perfectly good foods like potatoes, chicken, and fish can be deep-fried and changed into a bad source of grease. This used fat is biologically dangerous because the heated oils pick up oxygen—partial burning—and become *lipid oxides*. Not only is the grease low in EFAs, because of the heat, but the lipid oxides are toxic in themselves. Some are carcinogens, and may be related to some of the types of cancer seen in industrialized countries. Grease was not a problem in your grandmother's kitchen, because you could taste it, and too much grease made food unpalatable. However, deep-fried foods taste good; large amounts of grease are masked by

---

* Autopsies on young American soliders in the Korean War showed, for the first time in history, advanced atherosclerosis in teenagers.

artificial flavors, stabilizers, sugar, and salt. (Another rich source of toxic lipid oxides is burned meat—all that's dark on charcoal-broiled steaks and burgers, for instance.)

The importance of these studies on pigs and monkeys is the clarification of which fats are truly dangerous—or unfriendly. *Trans*-fat was the most damaging to the pig arteries; next most dangerous was grease. Neither of these fats is "natural": *trans*-fat results from hydrogenation, an industrial process; and grease results from heating and oxidizing fats. Natural food chains do not include this type of hydrogenation or oxidation, and therefore we do not have enzyme systems to handle the resultant toxic "unfriendly" fats.

The safest fats in this pig study were found in whole eggs and whole milk. Their natural content of EFAs probably made them a useful food for pigs. A little disease was caused by beef tallow and egg yolks, but both of these items can be considered somewhat processed since the protein of the beef and egg white had been removed. Fat should be "covered" by protein in the diet because fat is used with protein in the body—the term *lipoprotein* is used for this complex of lipids (fats) and proteins as it appears in our blood. Any diet that has too much fat will cause some disease simply because the excess fat cannot be used in the absence of protein.

WHAT KIND OF FAT DOES YOUR BODY HAVE? PUT IT DOWN ON PAPER!

You can estimate what kind of fat you have on your body if you write down the types of food you eat. If you have been eating the same sorts of foods for six years or longer, this is a very accurate method of classifying body fat. It is important to do this before you try to lose weight, because your expectations depend on how "friendly" your fat happens to be. It takes no special willpower to remove truly friendly fat; it just melts away with a little easy fasting. It is designed to do that. Its high EFA content makes it useful for energy. However, the low-EFA *"unfriendly" fat is dangerous and hard to lose!*

When you classify your fat intake, keep the very unfriendly *trans*-fat and lipid oxides separated from the saturated fats. The latter are only "slightly unfriendly."

Very Unfriendly Fat
1. *Trans*-fat, including all hydrogenated vegetable oils, those in margarine, cooking fats, shortening, plus those in processed foods. Read labels!
2. Toxic lipid oxides, or grease from frying and deep-frying. Most fast-food items have to be included here if they are deep-fried. Charbroiled steaks have black areas rich in lipid oxides.

Slightly Unfriendly Fat
1. Processed fats with EFAs removed, including powdered eggs (found in packaged items listing "egg" on the label), lard (used as shortening), and tallow. The latter are referred to as "animal fats."
2. Slightly processed fats with protein removed, including egg yolks (eaten without the protein of the whites), butter (with milk protein removed), and liquid vegetable oils (with the solid parts of the nuts and seeds removed).

Friendly Fat
The fats from whole foods such as whole milk, whole eggs, seeds, nuts, and whole grains. These vital fats come with a natural amount of EFAs, protein, and vitamin E. If your body fat is made from these sources, it is "friendly" and can be removed quickly with any kind of caloric restriction or any increase in physical exercise. No special willpower is needed, and there is no danger in this type of weight loss. Vegetarians who eat much of their meals raw or only slightly cooked will have this type of fat. The use of milk and eggs does not change it; many population studies support the idea that this type of eating—ovo-lacto-vegetarianism—is conducive to a long, healthy life.

After you have totaled your daily intake of each of these three kinds of fat, you must, if you are a smoker, make one major adjustment. This is the reason why the emphasis on the danger of smoking has shifted from cancer to heart disease.

But Smoking Makes All Fat Unfriendly!

Tobacco smoke contains many *oxides*—biologically active molecules which damage EFAs. Vitamin E is an *antioxidant* and can protect us from small amounts of carbon monoxide in a smoggy atmosphere; but if you are actually smoking yourself, the burden of oxidants coming into your body is too high for dietary vitamin E to handle. Polyunsaturates are very delicate molecules, and it is hard to protect them in tissue. The antioxidants vitamin E and vitamin C are important protective molecules, but they cannot protect a smoker. If you are a smoker, consider all of your body fat to be "unfriendly" in the lipid-oxide group.

VISUALIZE THE FAT ON YOUR BODY BY POURING IT OUT IN THE KITCHEN

Let us assume that you are twelve pounds too heavy. You look into the mirror, recalling what you looked like in high school, and you see a surplus of about twelve pounds of fat. That is about twelve pints—six quarts of fat! Go out to the kitchen and find twelve pint-sized containers—jars of peanut butter, mayonnaise, or shortening. Try to get a mixture of containers that fits the proportion of each type of fat in your diet: greasy drippings from frying, butter or margarine, liquid vegetable oils, cream, and eggs. When you actually look at twelve pounds of dietary fat, you will see the biological chore you have set out for yourself in losing weight!

Lard will make up over half the fat, since we make lard out of all extra calories that do not burn with exercise. Seven pint cans of lard! A lot of calories—about 24,000 of them, the energy equivalent of walking 240 miles. It's buried in your body.

Vegetable oils cannot make up more than a third of your

fat, because that is about the limit of polyunsaturates any animal can store from a vegetarian diet. Three pints of corn oil is a reasonable amount the average person might be carrying around. Remember, this is slightly unfriendly fat—and it will require about the same expenditure of calories per pint to remove as lard.

I assume you do not smoke. This would leave the oil in a biologically friendly state—ready to burn for energy when needed. If you do smoke, you will have to imagine that the oil has turned rancid (oxidized) and will make you sick and weak when you try to burn it for energy. This is why joggers stop smoking—their bodies tell them to!

The remaining two pounds of fat will be either butter, cream, and eggs (if you are a careful eater), or grease, margarine, and rancid fat (if you are a fast-food eater). The more friendly this fat mixture, the easier your weight loss will be. But note that the friendly fat is still only a small part of the fat you intend to lose.

Predict How Much Will Be Water Loss

"The first seven pounds don't count." This is a simple rule for judging the success of a weight-loss program. About seven pounds of water are "available" for weight loss before body fat is lost. This includes: salt water, glycogen water, gut water, sweat, and muscle water. Not *all* of your body water will be lost, of course, but some will go at the start of a diet.

Salt Water—The amount of body water is proportional to the amount of sodium (Na) in the body. If you add salt (sodium chloride, NaCl) to your food for a few days, you can gain about two pounds of water. If you go on a low-salt diet for five days, your kidneys will dump about two pounds of body water. A high-fiber diet keeps the body from absorbing some of the salt, so just adding cereal bran to your meals may take these two pounds of salt water off.

Glycogen Water—The fuel stored in your muscles for short, fast exercise is a carbohydrate called *glycogen*. The molecule looks something like the starch molecule, and it is surrounded by water molecules. Athletes can easily store up two pounds of this glycogen-water mixture. After exercise, about twelve miles of walking or jogging, the fuel will be gone, along with the water. (Walking is less strenuous than running, but the amount of glycogen you burn also depends on your exercise level. So we may consider twelve miles for a *walker* to be roughly equivalent to twelve miles for a *runner*.)

Gut Water—Several bulky meals can easily weigh two pounds. It will take many hours for your body to extract the gut water and get rid of it. If you change from a high-residue diet to a low-residue diet you may easily drop two pounds of gut water.

Sweat—The usual sweat loss during vigorous exercise is two pounds per hour. If it is warm you lose more; in cool weather you lose less. A steam room can also take off pounds of sweat. As we will see, a dangerous idea!

Muscle Water—After several hours of vigorous exercise, the involved muscle groups will appear larger due to a normal swelling that is associated with the increased metabolic activity and heat. A fifteen-mile walk can leave two pounds of "muscle water" in your legs for almost a whole day. This phenomenon thus often balances sweat loss.

How to Lose Eight Pounds in a Day—For Nothing!

If you eat several high-carbohydrate meals and stop exercising for a couple of days, your body will take on two pounds of glycogen and water. Let's assume that you weigh 175 pounds at this time. Then you fast overnight and walk for four hours at dawn. You use up the glycogen and sweat off two more pounds of water. Total weight loss is four pounds; you now weigh 171 pounds. Now you start to restrict salt intake and go on a low-residue diet. Your weight goes back up to 173 as you drink to replace your sweat loss, but the gut water and the salt water start coming off—two pounds of each. So you drop from 173 to 169 with this four pounds of water loss.

Now you can try the sweat loss again: walking four hours and dropping from 169 to 167 pounds. Notice the wide range of body weight:

175 pounds—glycogen-loaded
173 pounds—resting weight
169 pounds—salt restriction and low-residue diet
167 pounds—sweat loss

Obviously, such water loss is temporary! It does not represent a true weigh loss.

This manipulation of body water is dangerous if carried too far. Steam rooms may raise your body temperature too high while squeezing out vital salts and minerals along with the sweat. Questionable weight-loss clinics may use diuretics (drugs that force the kidney to squeeze excess water out of your blood). The use of drugs and external heat is hazardous, and has no place in a sensible weight-control program. Your kidneys must control important salts in your body. If drugs confuse your kidney function, death can result when salt concentrations fluctuate too wildly.

ALL ROADS TO WEIGHT LOSS
LEAD TO "FASTING"!

In the best sense of the word, *fasting* is cutting something out of your ordinary diet. Unfortunately, fasting has religious overtones, yet even in the Christian churches the word is understood to mean simply a denial of full portions at certain meals—not eating just bread and water or water alone! As I have said, and as all responsible diet-promoters recognize, weight loss results only from a caloric deficit: you burn more calories than you ingest. There is no magic food that "melts fat away" or "burns excess fat" in your body. As we have seen, water loss is the most elusive factor in any diet; it's *fat* loss that counts.

So we must now consider how much you can cut back on your regular eating habits—from a little to all the way! Safely. Realistically. Building health rather than losing health with weight.

Does it make any difference whether you cut meals out, or cut back on each meal, or spread your intake over more, smaller meals, adding up to a deficit? It's commonly believed that dinner adds more weight to your body because "you can't work it off" before going to sleep. There's some truth to that idea. I'd rather put it this way: If you're going to eat a big meal, why waste it on a time when you have *other* ways to stave off hunger? Namely, sleep. You can't get hungry or eat while sleeping. But if you eat that big meal in the morning, your body will tell you not to eat again for some time.

Many dietary "tricks," as we will see in the next chapter, are based on just this principle: letting your body do your thinking for you. For example, the recent *Fabulous Fructose Diet* of Dr. J. T. Cooper is based on avoiding the "glucose-insulin trap," in which sugars fool the body into prematurely lowering the *blood* sugar, thus setting off appetite howls. Modern life has surrounded us with a multitude of such deceptive sugars. Dr. Cooper points out that only fructose, among the sugars, is "honest."

TWO FASTS

The Total Fast

This is a "water-only" fast—leaving you with a caloric deficit of about 1,500 calories a day (more if you are more active). However, the total fast should *not* be used for weight loss, since you are left with both a *calorie* deficit and a *nutrient* deficit. You lose fitness as you lose weight; and the calories are put back on with the nutrients as you replace them. Weight loss during a total fast removes 1,500 calories of body fat with EFAs, protein, and vitamins (nutrient removed from living cells to make up that day's nutrient requirements). Proper weight loss should not cause the loss of essential nutrients.

The Modified Fast

This fast uses low-calorie, high-nutrient supplements along with vigorous exercise. If walking is "vigorous" for you, then you walk three times a day—keeping a mileage diary along with a food diary. We will start simple, with a six-hour fast and a twenty-minute walk, just to give you some idea what you are about to undertake. *Remember, a mile is a hundred calories, whether you walk, jog, or run.* Speed isn't important; distance is.

Weight loss can be calculated on the basis of one pound of fat for each 3,500 calories deficit. I have seen many individuals lose a pound a week for a total of fifty pounds in a year. I have personally tried to test the maximum rate of weight loss for a month and managed to lose twenty-two pounds in thirty days. But this type of weight loss is very dangerous, and I will discuss the dangers before I discuss the actual details of the diet.

HAZARDS OF WEIGHT LOSS

Sudden Death

This has been reported as a result of unsupervised "liquid protein" diets. These diets are designed to be used under medical supervision; and even then are only used in cases of serious obesity. The reasons for these sudden deaths are many, and poorly understood.

The liquid protein used in the diet is not of good quality; usually it is industrial-grade protein hydrolysate that lacks one or more of the essential amino acids of which protein is made. Although the diet is supplemented with vitamins and minerals, none of this is in the form of raw, whole foods with natural nutrients. People on these diets put their bodies under severe nutritional stress, and they have to place too much trust in the scientists who design the diets and monitor their health.

The autopsies on these sudden deaths occasionally show *myocarditis* (an inflammation of the heart), but frequently nothing unusual is found. The heart just stops. I think the cause is a distortion of body chemistry caused by the diet.

I would never advise anyone to try a liquid protein diet for weight loss. Physicians who do advise it are careful to point out the hazards, and they use it only when there are strong reasons for it. Again, these diets should be used only under a doctor's care.

Kidney Stones

These can form during weight loss for several reasons. If fluids are restricted too much in an effort to avoid the calories they contain, urine output will drop off. But tissues break down during weight loss, putting an extra burden on the kidneys, which must excrete more material into the urine. Therefore, urine output should be *increased* during fasting.

The types of stones can vary. *Calcium stones* form during bone loss—and bone loss goes with weight loss. *Uric acid stones* are most often seen in gout patients, but uric acid increases during tissue breakdown. The pure *dehydration stone* is not really a stone at all; it is just a painful concentration of chemicals—phosphates or urates—that are normally present in the urine. If the body is dehydrated, crystals of these chemicals precipitate out of the urine.

Stones can be prevented if you produce a quart of clear urine each day. Cloudy or colored urine does not count! You must increase your fluid intake until you reach that goal. Herb teas and beer are good fluid sources. Tea has no calories, but beer has. Alfalfa tea and beer are also good sources of silicon (the fiber factor) and will help bring your tissue level of this vital nutrient up.

Constipation

A "low-fiber" disease. During fasting, your usual sources of food fiber may be bypassed to avoid calories. Cereal bran, alfalfa, and pectin should be taken to protect the gut. All contain silicon. It is important to keep the gut normal, not only to avoid hemorrhoids, but also to protect gut bacteria—"normal flora."

Stress

More dangerous during fasting. If your body becomes low in the water-soluble vitamins—B complex and C—then you are a candidate for "the virus." Flu symptoms appear in those who push their fasting too far. The virus is all around us; there are over thirty different strains, and they cause symptoms when you are weak and vulnerable.

Brewer's yeast, yogurt, and wheat germ are good sources of the B-complex vitamins. Fresh fruit and ascorbic-acid tablets are good sources of vitamin C.

Protein Loss

Result: weakness or ugliness, depending on where your body "cannibalizes" the essential amino acids it needs during fasting. No one wants to lose facial tissues to the point of looking cadaverous, and no one wants shoulder and arm muscles to waste away.

Protein can be spared during fasting if the essential amino acids are supplied each day. Good sources are brewer's yeast and wheat germ.

Smoking

Smokers can expect greater problems. Tobacco smoke contains oxidants that can destroy the antioxidants in the body—vitamins C and E.

Vitamin C protects you from stress and helps you build strong collagen—the stuff that knee joints and tendons are made of. Without vitamin C you cannot progress in an exercise program because your tendons and knee joints will always hurt, and the stress of heavy exercise will break you down, causing flu-like symptoms.

Without vitamin E your polyunsaturates will become toxic oxides, so your fatty fuel will be of poor quality—not available for energy. So without vitamin E you can't keep your strength up during fasting because you can't utilize your stored fat for fuel.

AVOIDING THE HAZARDS—WITH A
SENSE OF HUMOR

A sense of humor is the best indication of good health and nutrition. If you can cut calories and still exercise with a sense of humor, your diet has adequate amounts of nutrients. As soon as your protein metabolism starts to break down important body proteins, you will lose your sense of humor. Weakness and inability to exercise signal a further loss of nutrients, usually the vitamin B complex. Don't try to increase your exercise while fasting; do the same amount you did *before* the fast.

Sense of humor, of course, is an intangible thing. We use the phrase loosely to describe a quality we like in our friends. But I mean this is a very strict, *serious* sense. The opposite is self-importance, persecution complex, distress, irascibility, boredom.

If you're grumpy now, improve your diet until you have a sense of humor before fasting. Yeast, yogurt, and wheat germ are good sources of the vitamin B complex, and should improve your outlook. Cut down on the "empty" calories. Switch from processed food to whole, raw foods until you feel like going out and getting more exercise.

Finally, do *not* use the modified fast unless you exercise. Without activity of some kind, you cannot monitor your nutrients. You can't trust any food supplements to supply adequate nutrients. Only your own body can tell you what is adequate for you. If you are sedentary, you should start a walking program *before* you take up serious efforts at weight loss. Even if you do not drop your body weight, the added exercise will make you fitter by changing pounds of fat into pounds of muscle. *If you do try fasting while you are sedentary, you will not know when you become deficient in a nutrient until you get a symptom—weakness, flu symptoms, or worse.*

THE MODIFIED-FAST PLAN

The Six-Hour "Fast"

An easy way to start. Pick a six-hour period in the day, say noon till supper. Avoid all processed food and tobacco during this period. Drink only alfalfa tea, using alfalfa tablets and boiling water, and eat a couple of pieces of raw fruit. Before supper walk twenty minutes. Try this each afternoon for a week, and keep a diary. The twenty-minute walk burns about a hundred calories, equal to the raw fruit and alfalfa tea—your first modified fast!

Now, things like alfalfa tea aren't usually available in the supermarket. Later we'll talk about alternatives. But if weight loss is important to you, you'll make a trip to a health-food store.

You will note that you are able to eat a normal lunch and

supper around the six-hour fast, but during the fast you break even—you take in about a hundred calories and exercise off the same amount with the twenty-minute walk. This step alone may prevent you from gaining weight with coffee breaks and afternoon snacks!

The Twelve-Hour Fast

Just as easy if you pick the twelve hours between supper and breakfast. You will sleep eight hours, drink alfalfa tea in the evening, and have a beer when you wake up. Then walk for forty-five minutes to burn off the calories in the beer. Eat a normal supper before the twelve-hour fast, and a normal breakfast afterward. During the modified fast, you take in 250 calories of beer and burn it off with a two-and-a-half-mile walk. Do this for another week. See how you feel. Try drinking the beer before bedtime and walking when you wake up. Same caloric balance, and the beer might help you sleep.

The Eighteen-Hour Fast

After you let your body experience the six- and twelve-hour fasts, the next step is to combine them. Eat your usual lunch (try to avoid processed foods as much as possible) and "fast" until supper with fruit and tea. Eat a sensible supper and fast until breakfast with a beer. Walk before each meal to burn up the fruit and beer calories. Keep your alfalfa tea and yeast tablets handy; take one tablet an hour when awake.

Now look at your day. You can only snack between breakfast and lunch. You walk before supper and breakfast. If you are not smoking, this three-mile-a-day program will be very adequate for a serious attempt at real weight loss. If you *are* smoking, the results may be disappointing.

You'll have to agree that so far the "fasting" I'm talking about is quite minimal. You might call it "snack fasting."

The One-Day Fast

This comes when you think you're used to the eighteen-hour fast. It is built around two hours of walking, which can be broken down into three or four separate walks if necessary. Try the one-day fast once a week at first. If it is easy, do it every other day for two or three days each week. However, you should review the hazards of fasting before you try the one-day fast, and take specific steps to avoid them *all*.

Principle: two hours of walking (about six miles) equal 600 calories. Nutrients should include everything needed to prevent complications—and yet not exceed the 600 calories. You still burn about 1,500 calories in a normal day's living (aside from the walking)—and that's where you lose the weight.

The one-day fast starts and ends with a meal, usually the evening meal. If the meal is not extra large, you will have a twenty-four-hour period in which your caloric intake will match your exercise, leaving you with a deficit of about 1,500 calories, which is equivalent to a bit less than half a pound of fat.

Here's how I see a good twenty-four-hour fast—your recipe for a day. (At the end of the chapter I'll go into more detail about the foods to accompany your fasts.)

Eat your usual supper. Use moderation with second helpings, have only a piece of fresh fruit for dessert. Start your twenty-four-hour diary.

Drink herb teas all evening and walk an hour before bedtime. Your supper will settle well, and provide calories for a restful sleep.

Wake up in the morning, drink a half-pint of beer, and walk for half an hour. Grind your seeds and alfalfa, mix with a little yogurt. Take yeast and alfalfa tablets to work or school. During the day eat a head of lettuce or a tomato with lemon juice and salt. Eat two pieces of fresh fruit and take a gram of vitamin C. Drink a cup of herb tea each hour with a yeast and an alfalfa tablet.

Walk a quarter of an hour in the afternoon; for a light snack, scramble an egg lightly.

Before supper walk another quarter-hour and then drink the other half-pint of beer. Watch your urine output. Make certain fluid intake keeps your urine clear. Watch your stools. Make certain the cereal bran and alfalfa leaves keep your stools bulky and floating.

End your twenty-four-hour diary at night. Count up the calories taken in and burned up. They should be nearly equal.
Eat a light supper—about twenty-six hours after the previous day's supper.

Yes, I've heard all the usual complaints. What? Bran, alfalfa, yogurt, herb tea? Ugh! But bear with me. Remember, I'm giving you the principles, the hard medicine. Add or subtract seeds and nuts. Experiment. Walk more or less each time you try the fast.

Now the good news: you've lost half a pound! Yes, your "day fast" should result in a real weight loss of eight ounces. Not much, but it's a loss, not a phony loss. And you've gained health at the same time.

Obviously, those who burn fat best can fast longest. If the modified fast includes adequate nutrients, then many of the calories can come from stored body fat—if that fat is "friendly." A simple way to predict the length of a modified fast is by using the distance you can cover on foot. If you can walk six miles, you can probably fast for a day. Those who have walked twelve miles recently can probably string two modified-fast days together each week. Marathon runners (who can jog twenty-six miles) can try the three-day fast. Forty-mile finishers can fast for a week.

The Two-Day Fast

Joggers who can handle six miles in the morning and evening will be able to "fast" for two days. Their twelve miles allow them to eat 1,200 calories—almost a regular diet! Write down the calories eaten, trying to include foods from each of the following groups:

Raw fruit—two pieces a day, and ascorbic-acid tablets
Raw vegetables—salads with lemon juice, no oils
Seeds, nuts, and grains—a "granola" you can trust
Yogurt or whole milk

Whole eggs (blend raw with orange juice or milk; or cook
lightly)
Beer and brewer's-yeast tablets
Alfalfa tea and alfalfa tablets, cereal bran

By spreading the food out over the whole day, you will always
have something in your stomach. An hourly cup of tea will
keep your hands busy. Yeast tablets keep you cheerful, and
alfalfa tablets put fiber in your gut. Cereal bran has few calories.

Stick to these ingredients and you'll be surprised how filling
and satisfying two days of "fasting" can be. Actually, you can
even ignore the calories if you don't fool yourself by eating two
eggs or drinking two beers when you're committed to one. There
just aren't that many calories here!

If a Two-Day Fast Works So Well, Why Not a Week or More?

For obvious reasons, there is a limit to the amount of weight
you can lose with safety. I said I once lost twenty-two pounds
in thirty days. How much of that was fat? If we use the rule
that "the first seven pounds don't count," we are left with a
fifteen-pound "real" weight loss in thirty days—about half a
pound a day. That is still a significant loss! But I have several
factors in my favor.

1. I was already a marathon runner; I knew that my body fat
   was high in EFAs and available for energy use.
2. I had been weighed underwater and knew I was a hefty 22
   percent fat before the loss—and dropped to about 9 percent
   fat after the loss. We know that 9 percent fat is about average for male marathoners, so I was in no danger there.
3. I was ready to quit at any time. If it had become difficult,
   I would have returned to my usual diet.
4. I continued my heavy training mileage—over ten miles per
   day—which allowed me extra calories to cover nutrients.
   Several times a week I ran between twenty and thirty miles
   in a single day—allowing me to eat over 2,000 calories and
   still lose half a pound per day.

Even so, what's safe? I should point out the hazards I worried about.

Sudden Death: Since I was only dropping from 22 percent fat to 9 percent fat I did not think I was taxing my system too much. Also, I used my daily training mileage and sense of humor to evaluate nutrient intake.

Other Risks: I watched for signs of dehydration, constipation, flu symptoms, weakness, and other complications of fasting; but since they are not "sudden," I thought I would have time to react after the first warning.

In retrospect, I think that the loss of only two pounds per week would have been adequate—and safer! Against the risks, I learned that a "fasting diet" can be sustained for long periods. And I began to incorporate some of my newfound dietary friends into my usual eating habits.

NOW THE ANSWERS

The questions asked at the beginning of the chapter can now be answered.

1. What is it about obesity that is dangerous?

When obesity is associated with malnutrition, it is dangerous. Body fat should be stored calories, available for future energy needs. However, if the fatty tissue is deficient in protein, essential fatty acids, vitamins, and other nutrients, it is dangerous. If the fat contains unnatural molecules—*trans*-fat or toxic lipid oxides—then these dangerous molecules can cause disease. If a person is obese, but not deficient, then he can be healthy.

2. How much weight loss is "true loss"?

This varies with the individual, but there are about seven pounds of extra body water than can be squeezed out before fat tissue is lost. Also, fat loss that is associated with nutrient loss will not benefit you, because the calories will have to be replaced as nutrients are replaced. Excess loss of nutrients is dangerous.

3. Why do some people stay thin while others put on a few pounds each year?

A refined diet has fewer nutrients, and extra calories must be taken in to satisfy nutrient needs. The extra calories add weight. Thin people get by because their choice of foods contains more nutrients. Smokers usually gain weight because the oxides in the smoke destroy EFAs in the diet. The resultant low-EFA fat is deficient and is difficult to burn with exercise or fasting, and thus it must be stored as extra body fat.

Someday I think it will be common knowledge that sugar, refined white flour, and cigarette smoke are all brothers under the skin. The first two are passive killers; the last is an active killer.

4. Is willpower important when cutting calories?

No, but common sense is. A menu high in nutrients will give you plenty of energy while you're cutting calories. "Empty calories" will be easy to skip. However, most foods must be eaten whole and raw in order to obtain maximum nutrients. This you must *know*.

5. Why is weight loss sometimes dangerous?

Deficiency in any vital nutrient can be dangerous. For this reason it is best to avoid all refined foods when cutting calories. Natural, whole, raw foods contain what *they* needed to live and grow; and if they are eaten this way, they supply us with what evolution designed *us* to live on. Sick people lose weight, but that's a poor reason to get sick.

6. How do you know that you are becoming healthier as you lose weight?

By exercise. If your daily exercise program becomes easier, then you are healthier. A better mix of nutrients helps, of course, but so does the lower body weight. Exercising without a sense of humor can be dangerous. As soon as your body gets into trouble and starts to burn protein, you will lose your sense of humor. Call this, if you will, the Bassler Inner-Smile Principle. It works!

OTHER QUESTIONS I'M OFTEN
ASKED ONLY IN PRIVATE

1. Why do I get uglier when I lose weight?

Protein loss from the face is a signal that you are trying to lose weight while deficient in a vital nutrient. Ugly fat stays on the belly and hips because it can't be burned for energy while you are deficient. First, improve nutrition so you can exercise better; then you are ready to cut calories!

2. If I lose weight, and live longer—will I *enjoy* it?

Yes, if you improve your nutrition and increase your exercise capability while you lose weight. Most "diseases of old age" are really deficiencies: EFAs, silicon, amino acids, vitamins, etc. Unfortunately, many people are fatalistic about their vices— they'd rather die at retirement age than face a nursing home. Overweight and "over-smoked" people perhaps don't want to enjoy their old age.

3. About those foods in a fasting diet—must I eat them?

I said at the beginning that once you understand the principles of weight loss you can create your own diet. Let's look at the foods again:

Beer will keep your urine output at a safe level. It also supplies silicon and some of the B vitamins. Take a pint for each six miles; and "cover" it with twelve of the 7½-grain brewer's yeast tablets.

Fresh fruit has water-soluble vitamin C and pectin, another source of silicon. Whole fruit is a living thing, and, as such, is a source of many nutrients. Also take a gram of ascorbic acid for each six miles.

Raw vegetables are also living things, rich in water-soluble vitamins and other nutrients. One tomato and one head of lettuce can be eaten with salt and lemon juice for a low-calorie meal.

Seeds and nuts are good sources of friendly fat and vitamin E if they are eaten whole and raw. Sunflower seeds can be chewed, but sesame seeds should be ground to a powder in a coffee mill before being eaten. (Use dry alfalfa leaves to keep the mill dry, otherwise you will have a paste similar to peanut butter.) Peanuts and pumpkin seeds are also easy to handle in a fast. Measure with a teaspoon; count calories!

The egg—one for each six miles. Scramble it in a pan with a little salt and pepper—a real treat during a fast.

Plain yogurt—about a fourth of a cup—is a good way to eat the seeds and nuts, or add it to the fresh fruit.

Cereal bran and alfalfa leaves can be taken as "tea" with boiling water, or mixed with yogurt, or swallowed as tablets— one an hour. Keep the fiber intake high enough to keep your stools bulky and floating.

There you have the principles behind my choices of food for a fasting diet. Now let's see what you can substitute on your own, based on the three key nutrients I mentioned earlier in this chapter: silicon, essential fatty acids, and antioxidants. Another way to remember them: foods with (1) crunch, (2) friendly fats, and (3) vitamin C.

On the fasting diet, substitute foods that supply one or more of the above three nutrients. Instead of beer, choose anything with silicon (remember crunch!). And drink plenty of water. Instead of tomato and lettuce or citrus fruits, substitute a potato for the vitamin C—or any of the darker-green leafy vegetables. For friendly fats, try cereal grains instead of seeds and nuts—or an additional egg. Note that where there's silicon, friendly fats, and vitamin C, there will also be, in order: the other minerals, protein, and the other vitamins. This, in a nutshell, is the basis for the Whole Life Diet. Now let's see how it can be applied to a wide variety of lifestyles and individual circumstances.

THREE

Tricks and Traps in Your Diet

I have a chess-playing friend who has devoted a good part of his leisure time to studying the principles of the game. He can quote the theorists if you ask him. He enjoys the logical analysis of any challenge—knowing the reason why. And yet he has told me that when it comes to the actual playing of a game he usually wins or loses because of some "trap."

I think the same thing is true in most practical situations, including sticking to a diet! Certainly it's clear to me that scientific research in the field of nutrition plods along on the evidence of one little study after another. Only after dozens, perhaps hundreds, of reports pile up do we see a pattern that we can rely on with any certainty. And the person trying to lose weight (and gain health) cannot be expected to remember the functions of the glands, the purposes of the various vitamins and minerals, or the good and bad points of various foods. What I find helpful is to read whatever I can that interests me—and let the unusual fact stand out. So to help you get a feel for the principles behind the statements in the previous chapter, I'd now like to show you some curious and interesting facts—some tricks and traps, if you will.

ALFALFA AND ARTHRITIS

Monkeys were protected from a high-cholesterol diet by alfalfa.[1] Butter was used as a source of fat, and the diet was followed with blood tests for cholesterol and other fats. Autopsies were done to show disease after six months. Some of the monkeys with disease were given a 50 percent alfalfa diet and the atherosclerosis regressed in six months. The level of fat intake was as high as the usual American diet during regression.

Alfalfa reduced the disease in rabbits fed sucrose and hydrogenated coconut oil.[2] (If you read the label on the cream substitute you use in your coffee, you will probably see "hydrogenated coconut oil." Then, if you add table sugar—sucrose—to the coffee, you are using the diet that caused atherosclerosis in rabbits.)

How does alfalfa protect against atherosclerosis?

Schwarz suggests that the active ingredient in food fiber is silicon, and alfalfa has 12,000 parts per million (ppm).[3] He suggests that a natural diet high in silicon may play a role in protecting against atherosclerosis, arthritis, and other degenerative diseases.

Schwarz checked out hair samples from cardiac athletes, champion athletes, and disabled patients to see if there was any relationship between disease and silicon.[4] Champions had normal levels (over 20 ppm), and some very low levels (under 4 ppm) were seen among patients with symptoms of atherosclerosis and/or arthritis. Patients taking alfalfa and other food fiber had elevated silicon levels (up to 100 ppm). Moral: Watch out for sucrose and "whitener" in your coffee, and think of alfalfa and other silicon sources as "protectors." There may also be help here for arthritis sufferers.

ASCORBIC ACID AND STRESS

The stress of a six-mile run can be compared to minor surgery. Patients have had their ascorbic-acid (vitamin C) levels checked, so I will use them as an example of minor stress.[5] Both major and minor surgery were followed by a 42 percent drop in blood ascorbic acid on the third day after the operation. This fits with the experience of some athletes who developed flu-like symptoms of stress on the third day after the race.

This suggests that extra vitamin C might be useful in handling stress.

BEER—IT'S MORE THAN WATER

"Moderate" beer drinking is associated with 50 percent protection against heart attacks.[6]

This same protection has been reported in the hard-water areas of Finland. The hard water was found to have twice the silicon as the soft water, and Schwarz suggests that it is the silicon that protects against heart attack.[7] Beer has 35 ppm silicon, while hard water has only 8 ppm!

"Moderate" alcohol intake was defined as 50 grams per day or 4 pints of brown ale—or 3 pints of mild draft beer.[8] The safety of ingesting 50 to 70 grams of ethanol per day is discussed by Howorth.[9]

Beer also contains potassium. And brewer's yeast can be used to "cover" the calories in beer with vitamin B complex.

The hazards of alcohol abuse begin with damage to the liver, but this usually happens when alcohol provides more than 40 percent of the calories.[10] *Any* refined calorie causes disease at this level of intake.

THE "PROTEIN" FAST:
AN OVERWEIGHT PERSON CAN
STARVE TO DEATH

Total fasting to lose weight is so dangerous that the editors of the *British Medical Journal* suggest that obesity should be handled in our schools through education, so proper eating and exercise patterns will be set in childhood.[11] They review the hazards of the total fast (water only) and the supplemented fast (synthetic nutrients without calories). The complications include sudden death, hair loss, bone loss, depression, weakness, muscle cramps, vomiting, sterility, loss of sex drive, and bad breath. For obvious reasons, they warn that fasting should not be a do-it-yourself project!

One of the supplemented fasts associated with sudden death is the so-called liquid protein diet discussed earlier, using an industrial-grade protein hydrolysate made from beef hides or collagen. The theory that protein loss from the body during fasting can be modified by adding something to the diet has given rise to a number of supplements to be taken when calories are reduced. Everyone agrees that man is not designed to live very long on a synthetic diet; but under certain conditions a patient's health is so threatened by obesity that supplemented fasting is prescribed.

One girl went on a liquid protein diet against her doctor's advice. She wanted to lose weight, but after dropping 120 pounds, she died! [12] Her diet was synthetic, and clearly deficient in many things.[13] Letters from several medical schools discussed the hazards of the liquid protein diet in the pages of the *New England Journal of Medicine*. Among the nutrients missed were some of the following: tryptophan (an amino acid), potassium, sodium, magnesium, copper, phosphate, selenium, vitamin E, and trace elements.

Moral: Raw, whole foods are safer than supplements! The autopsy on the girl who lost 120 pounds showed the cardiac effects of "starvation" in spite of the fact that she was still obese. This supports my view that the body will take what it needs from living cells if the stored fatty tissue is not "burnable"—if the fat is "unfriendly" and will not supply needed energy. Obese people who fast too long can use up nutrients and *starve while still obese!*

Human-Autopsy Studies of Fatty Acids

Americans eat more saturated fats than the Japanese, and their body fat is more saturated.[14] Americans have more coronary heart disease and less tissue linoleic acid—the important essential fatty acid. As compared to the Japanese, Americans have 6 percent less linoleic, 5 percent more oleic, and 2 percent more stearic fatty acid.

During severe weight loss, Japanese men lose linoleic acid first, and the resultant mixture of fatty acids was lower in this essential fatty acid, giving them an "unfriendly fat" pattern that was more like the Americans'. Other studies also show less coronary heart disease with high linoleic levels.[15]

SUGAR—A HAZARDOUS SUBSTANCE

As an "empty calorie," sugar is something like alcohol *to all people:* it gives us calories without nutrients, so we wind up with a deficiency of nutrients. That means either of two things: (1) if we overeat to get the absent nutrients, we become overweight; (2) if we don't overeat, we become undernourished and prone to illness and disease.

Second, sugar embodies the danger of any carbohydrate eaten in excess: it creates *saturated* fat in the body. If you eat unsaturated fat, the resultant body fat can be very unsaturated also.[16] If that fat is stored in your body as unburned, excess fat, it's safer in that form than in saturated form. But all excess calories from carbohydrates increase fat synthesis in the body— and fat synthesized in the body is only *saturated*. Animals fed glucose or fructose after a preceding fast produced the most massive synthesis of fatty acids.[17] Naturally, it's better not to overeat at all—but when you do, *sugars* (and other carbohydrates) are worse for your body than fats.

Third, a more serious and the most popularized danger of sugar in the diet is functional hypoglycemia (see Chapter Four). It's worth pointing out that one of the sugars, fructose in pure form, apparently avoids the glucose-insulin trap.

Small amounts of sugar, especially in the form of fruits or honey, can't be dangerous. Many nutrients are "acting in harmony" with the sugar in this form.

I believe that the least recognized danger of refined sugar is its "masking" effect on our palates. There's so much of it in our foods that we can't hear what those foods are trying to tell us, so we can't rely on our natural cravings to guide us to the right foods.

STEWS AND STEAKS—THE ONION
AND GARLIC BELONG

Carnitine, a B vitamin found in meats, transports fatty acids into cells where they are burned for energy. Carnitine helps you burn fat! Our muscle cells have carnitine in high levels. During starvation there is a choice between fat and muscle when the body is searching for calories. If a muscle cell is damaged, it releases carnitine into the system. This signals the body to burn fat. Thus, nature has provided muscle cells with a tool to defend themselves against being used for fuel during starvation. The carnitine they release actually helps the body to burn fat.[18]

Therefore, it would be logical to use beef stew during a modified fast. Stew contains rich amounts of carnitine, all the amino acids, salt, fluids, fat, and very few calories. Since it is low in carbohydrates, it would permit the body to continue to burn fat during the fast.

Beef is not intrinsically bad, but it can be turned into a dangerous food in several ways.

Range-fed steers obtain rich amounts of natural fats in their grazing. Since they eat living vegetable material, their intake of essential fatty acids (EFAs) and vitamin E is adequate. This is reflected in their meat. The carcass has less fat, and a higher level of EFA. However, feed lots are used to fatten cattle with old grain—a poor source of EFA. They get less exercise and gain more weight. Hormones and antibiotics also help them grow faster. When they come to market they are actually obese—up to 80 percent of the "meat" calories can be fat due to marbling. There is more fat to the cut and it is lower in EFA. Of course, it is more tender, has more flavor, and is more profitable to produce. Unfortunately, it is also more dangerous to eat!

After the beef gets into your kitchen, you can improve it or make it more dangerous, depending on how you prepare it. The saturated fat in the cut is probably low in EFAs. This is not too important if you just use a quarter of a pound per person to flavor your vegetable soup. Excess fat comes to the top and can be skimmed off. However, if you charbroil it, you can form toxic lipid oxides when the meat turns black on the surface.

Onions can be used to cancel out the effect of steak on your blood cholesterol. If you eat your steak "smothered in onions," you will be happy to know that animal studies have shown that onions and garlic actually removed some of the atherosclerosis caused by a high-fat diet. Human studies showed that onions or garlic will lower the serum cholesterol of those on a high-fat diet.[19] Each human was given about a stick of butter and the cholesterol rose about 10 percent. However, when onion and butter were given together, the cholesterol actually went *down* about 3 percent!

How much onion do you need?

Each ounce of onion protects you from two ounces of butter. Since butter is a saturated animal fat, this ratio of onion to fat would be about the same for a steak. If you eat a pound of steak that is 50 percent fat, you are getting half a pound of fat and will need a quarter of a pound of onion with it. That would be a steak "smothered in onions"! This may be a biological explanation for the extensive use of garlic and onions in otherwise fatty or oily recipes. The "essential oils" of onion and garlic protect you from the fats in meat sauces and salad dressings. This protection translates into improved flavor, because the fats and oils are metabolized more efficiently.

HAZARDS OF REFINED POLYUNSAT-URATES—BUTTER REALLY IS BETTER

Synthetic diets containing polyunsaturated fats shortened the life of mice. Lard was safer. Both diets contained 20 percent fat.[20] The *mean* life span was shortened from 29.3 months on lard to 24.3 months for safflower oil—a 5-month drop, about a sixth! The reason for the drop is the presence of toxic *free radicals* formed by oxygen reacting with the double bonds of the unsaturated fatty acids.

Another way to look at it is a deficiency in the antioxidants, vitamins C and E, which would prevent the oxygen from reacting with the fatty acids. Thus, the safflower oil was not protected from oxidants. Any synthetic diet would have this same hazard. The authors suggest that toxic free radicals make the human use of polyunsaturated fats suspect. I agree. There is a possibility that cancer is increased when polyunsaturates are added to diets.[21] It is safer to eat whole foods, mostly raw.

UNFRIENDLY FATS: WATCH THAT PEANUT-BUTTER-AND-MARGARINE SANDWICH!

Much of the literature on unfriendly fats can be traced to Dr. George Mann of Vanderbilt University and Dr. Fred Kummerow of the University of Illinois at Urbana. Of course, they do not use the term "unfriendly fats" in their publications, but they do clearly show that some dietary fats are biologically hazardous while others are actually good for you.

Kummerow's work with pigs clearly points out that margarines with *trans*-fat cause vascular disease much more easily than natural fats in whole eggs and whole milk.[22]

Mann's writings have pointed out that much of the diet information available to the public has been unscientific—and based on industrial and political interests rather than basic research.[23] He suggests that a low-cholesterol, low-fat, polyunsaturated-fat diet may *not* be the answer in treatment of coronary heart disease. He showed that *whole* milk actually lowers blood cholesterol levels.[24] He agrees that the margarines have dangerous *trans*-fats resulting from hydrogenation.[25]

Kummerow showed that *trans*-fat caused disease even in the presence of adequate essential fatty acids.[26]

Imai worked with toxic lipid oxides and produced damage in artery walls—in only twenty-four hours![27]

Fats that have been burned (lipid oxides) and hydrogenated (*trans*-fat) are very unfriendly. Just how unfriendly can be seen when *trans*-fat is compared to essential fatty acids in monkeys.

We all eat bread with shortening. Just how critical is the

degree of hydrogenation of this shortening? The monkey study needed only five months to cause atherosclerosis and five months to remove it. The diet was 40 percent fat, and the fat was hidden in the whole-wheat bread. Nothing else in the diet was changed.[28] When the bread contained hydrogenated peanut butter, disease progressed. This diet contained *trans*-fat, which is unnatural. When the bread contained liquid safflower oil, the disease regressed; and the arteries recovered. Both diets were 40 percent fat, but safflower oil is high in essential fatty acids (EFAs).

Monkeys are like us in many ways; and five months is a very short time. So I think we should worry about the type of shortening in our bread. Every meal counts!

Analysis of ninety-two brands of margarine and eighteen brands of shortening showed that *none* was completely free of dangerous *trans*-fatty acids.[29]

THE GIANT MEAL—IS IT DANGEROUS?

A physician-marathoner in his mid-forties spent five hours in a restaurant entertaining friends. Afterward, he weighed five pounds more and did not feel like jogging. During the evening he had consumed five bottles of beer, a platter of salty corn chips with dip, prime rib, shrimp, baked potato, salad, rice, carrots, bread and butter, coffee, and mushroom "in a skillet."

Why did he gain five pounds?

Salt. The meal included a massive supply of table salt hidden in the chips, chip dip, salad dressing, vegetables, and the various sauces used for the meat and shrimp. Two pounds of body water would be held by salt; two pounds of gut water would be held by the bulk of the meal, and the dry weight of the food plus the fat would be another pound.

What made him not feel like running?

There are three reasons why a meal like that would make a marathoner feel sluggish. The *bulk* of such a large meal can elevate the diaphragm, making running uncomfortable. The *type of fat* is wrong for running. Too much saturated fat in the beef, fried shrimp, butter, and sauces; too much *trans*-fat in the shortening in the bread and chips; and possibly too much grease or lipid oxides. The *amount* of fat may have exceeded his tolerance. Most marathon runners eat a high-carbohydrate diet and develop a fatty-food intolerance. Excess fat in the diet causes gastric distention—a sensation of "fullness."

Is the meal dangerous?

It depends on the caloric intake for the rest of the day and the total exercise. Such a large meal can be balanced by a ten-mile run and twelve hours of fasting. However, for a sedentary person to eat this way could cause trouble. Those with hypertension would get too much salt. Those with coronary heart disease would get too much fat. An obese person would get too many calories.

Moral: Only adequate exercise may protect you from a food binge.

EXERCISE: IT DOES MORE THAN BURN CALORIES OR BUILD MUSCLES!

Dr. George Mann suggests that exercise will help protect body protein from loss during fasting.[30] When you are losing weight, the body can take nutrients from either protein or fat; but if you are exercising vigorously, the body is more likely to spare protein and burn the fat if it can. You must exercise to keep your muscles and bones strong during fasting; otherwise you will become weak due to loss of protein.

Moral: If you use it, you won't lose it! Use your muscles and bones every day and you won't lose them during fasting.

Actually, Mann suggests that exercise is a healthier way to lost weight than cutting calories. I think that everyone would agree with that! The objection we always hear is how many miles you have to run to "make up" for a martini (one and a half) or a chocolate almond bar (three). The answer to that is exercise *allows* you to fast safely, and *tells* you when it isn't safe!

ALCOHOL, EXERCISE, AND SEX—
NOT IN THAT ORDER!

There are many reports that sexual performance is improved, at least in the male, by fasting! More on other aspects of diet and sex later. The theory is based on the priorities that various functions of the body have. The brain makes the first demands on the available supply of oxygen, then the cardiovascular system, and so forth down the line. Last on the list are the sexual organs. But when fasting reduces the demands of the "higher" systems, the gonads receive more of the benefits of the blood. Similarly, when the pituitary function is depressed by poor diet, "the sex hormones are always the first affected" in the "order of sacrifice" postulated by K. J. Franklin.

The other side of the coin is that the male hormone testosterone is produced in significantly lower quantities for eight hours or more after strenuous exercise, according to Dr. Rex Wiederanders. And the depressant effects of alcohol are well known.

But there's an escape clause for beer and wine! Dr. Carl C. Pfeiffer writes, in *Mental and Elemental Nutrients,* his classic study of orthomolecular medicine:

> Sexual performance is enhanced by beer or pleasant wine at dinner, but it is inhibited by strong empty-calorie beverages such as liquors and mixed drinks. You may want to plan an intimate dinner for two; serve wine; and in place of dessert approach your companion and say, "I'm on a strict diet and need to burn off 400 calories tonight!"[31]

Moral: You can do some things on an empty stomach, but not on empty calories.

FOUR

Find Your Bodyprint– And Use It!

Two young women stand before me—young, slim, glowing with the flush of a vigorous life. They've just finished a ten-kilometer run, six miles through the park on an early spring morning. I congratulate them on their times; I've watched them progress from self-conscious, timid teenagers to self-confident athletes. They're so much alike they even make a point of crossing the finish line together. And I'm about to make a mistake that doctors and the general public alike are so prone to make in comparing two people.

I'm about to assume these two young people are just about the same *beneath* their skin as they are on the surface.

Wrong. There's nothing mysterious about it. Sure, they are individuals in their feelings, sensibilities, psyches. That's a truism of our individualistic age. But they're also quite different in a very measurable way. Biologically, they can be miles apart—even though they may be the same age, have the same build, similar backgrounds, and similar diets and exercise. Their internal chemistry has stamped each of them with a *bodyprint* that is as unique as a fingerprint. Only, unlike a fingerprint, a bodyprint can be *grossly* different from one person to the next.

Medical science has acknowledged this fact with its head, but hasn't accepted it with its heart. "Biochemical individuality" has been demonstrated since the late nineteenth century, but doctors and researchers go on acting as if (1) there is a single ideal chemical composition of our bodies, and (2) a person with no overt signs of illness can be assumed to have a "healthy" chemical balance. Neither is true.

General appearances help to perpetuate both assumptions. True, we can see that the body of a sprinter is obviously different from the body of a long-distance runner. Indeed, their differing musculatures and heartbeats can tell us something about their biochemical selves. An obese person is likely to have a cardiovascular system quite unlike that of an active person. But beyond these gross indications, general appearances tell us virtually nothing about the functions of the body's various glands, its metabolism, or the quality of its blood.

Even the familiar measurements of pulse, temperature, and blood pressure no longer are tied to a fixed standard—a standard that marks the "normal" person. Just a few years ago, if you went to a blood bank to give your bimonthly pint and registered a pulse rate of 60, you would have been sent home. Now they ask you pleasantly, "Are you a runner?" Once, the marathon runner Ron Wayne happened to be sitting next to an eminent heart specialist at a banquet, when the subject of pulse rates came up. Ron casually mentioned that his was about 30. "Nonsense!" scoffed the doctor. "If you showed up in my office with that heartbeat, I'd rush you to a hospital." Ron offered his wrist to the doctor; true to form, the medical Neanderthal refused to take his pulse!

But, you say, blood pressure *is* a gold standard of sorts—120 over 80 is the ideal of the teenager, and the closer we get to that the better. Perhaps.

And how about cholesterol? We know that a high level is associated with atherosclerosis. Or do we?

HEALTH ISN'T A PLACE—
IT'S A DIRECTION

The first organized study of the phenomenon of individual biochemical differences has been carried on for more than ten years now at the Institute of Health Research, a small but trend-setting nonprofit firm in San Francisco. Here, under the direction of Dr. George Zur Williams, several thousand men and women of all ages have undergone a series of blood tests each year to establish their own bodyprints. As Dr. Williams says, they are finding out what their own ideal standards are, so that in succeeding years they can detect a movement away from those guidelines.

The institute concedes that a cholesterol reading of 210 milligrams per deciliter of blood is statistically a good indication that the arteries aren't likely to form the plaques that characterize atherosclerosis. But a reading of 300 may be acceptable for one person's biochemical individuality, while a reading of 200 might not fit well at all with another's. And this is only one example— a highly visible example, to be sure—of what it means to have "ideal" standards of one's own.

To take full advantage of Dr. Williams's program, your first year of blood tests must coincide with a period in your life when you can attest to being healthy. Ideally, that's when you're young, or getting back in shape after the usual excesses of middle age. Thereafter, any small change in any of the twenty-three variables tested can indicate a direction, an incipient health problem.

How do you know when you're "feeling good"? Nobody can tell you better than yourself. The institute uses a complex questionnaire, computerized and analyzed against the profile of a "healthy population." But you must look into yourself and your recent past to come up with the answers. In the absence of any overt problems, it's enough if you can honestly say you're handling your work and your leisure effectively. Even if you're sixty or older, the health profile you project at that age may be of inestimable value in seeing how you are *moving* over the next decade or two.

HEALTHY UNTIL PROVEN SICK?

In this country we're legally innocent until proven guilty. By an unfortunate analogy, medical practice commonly assumes people are healthy until proven sick—and then the treatment begins. Not that preventive medicine isn't all the rage; we see pious statements every day about striving for optimum health instead of simply avoiding sickness. That's all to the good, but according to Dr. Williams it's not good enough. He grew up in a remote part of China where doctors were paid only when the villagers were healthy, instead of when they had to be treated. Many years later, as director of clinical pathology for the National Institutes of Health, he became more and more concerned with the flight of research dollars almost exclusively into detection and treatment of disease. In 1969 he finally got the chance to establish an institute devoted to the detection of *subclinical* disease. And therein is the difference between what is bandied about as "preventive medicine" and what he calls "health watch."

A thorough medical checkup—the well-known "annual"—can and does detect the early form of a disease—a disease in progress. Dr. Williams maintains that only a minute examination of your "bodyprint" from year to year can turn up the conditions *underlying* a disease. In the early years of the Institute of Health Research, several profiles showed a drastic change in the level of liver enzymes. But, when contacted, these individuals assured the institute that they were feeling fine. Dr. Williams pursued their cases and later discovered that they were all suffering from subclinical hepatitis. This and many other underlying conditions may be quite prevalent in the general population—only the national expansion of "health watch" can determine with reliability. But for now Dr. Williams is content to conclude, "Few people have any realistic idea of just what degree of health they do enjoy."

All of this is wonderful, you say. But what if I don't live in

San Francisco, and an institute like Dr. Williams's never comes my way? Well, you may not be able to analyze a blood workup, and compare one year's to the next. But you *can* avail yourself of many other kinds of physical testing. You *can* watch key indicators, such as triglycerides and cholesterol. And you *can* carry on a dialogue with your physician about your level of health, instead of simply nodding your head as he tells you to lose some weight and get some exercise. For now you know that *you are not like anybody else.*

TESTING, TESTING . . .

The most common way nowadays to find out more about yourself—that hidden *you* beneath your skin—is to sign up for a physical-fitness exam. Many YMCAs around the country offer such a program in conjunction with a local hospital. Several commercial firms, such as Fitness Centers of America and Vital Fitness Evaluation Centers, now offer their services in major cities. And various universities and community hospitals have excellent programs involving treadmill tests, determinaton of body fat, and measurement of oxygen capacity and uptake. More on all of these in a minute. It should be pointed out that the aerobics generation has spawned something more than running-shoe stores and gigantic marathons. The medical industry has also responded to the demands of this new health-conscious breed.

An excellent example is the alertness of a laboratory testing firm, MetPath, in seeing the importance of high-density lipoprotein (HDL) in the composition of cholesterol. The general public is still being bombarded with the notion that a high cholesterol reading is the danger sign—now many years after it has been shown conclusively that HDL, which may account for a high proportion of serum cholesterol, actually protects against coronary heart disease (CHD). In a newsletter sent to psysicians in mid-1977, MetPath offered a complete update on the relationship between HDL and CHD. The firm was attempting to point out its ability to test for HDL, and naturally wished to convince doctors of the importance of that test for their patients. MetPath paraphrased an admonition from Dr. Donald S. Frederickson, Director of the National Institutes of Health:

   . . . before a person found to have high blood cholesterol is placed on a stringent low-cholesterol diet or treated with cholesterol-lowering drugs, analysis should be made of his HDL. If high HDL is what accounts for most of his cholesterol, then treatment may be unnecessary or undesirable.[1]

How can you, as a layman, know about such things when all you hear in the daily press is the chant against cholesterol, and food cholesterol at that! Fortunately, the gap between the informed layman and the medical profession has been narrowed considerably by the impact of the aerobics generation. The common ground between doctors and exercise-conscious people even has a new name: sports medicine. Whereas once our doctors—and our culture—would say to a sick person, "Lie down," nowadays *rest* is not taken for granted as the answer to every unspecific health problem. The dangers of trying to "run through" pain or stress have also been broadcast. Yet it is the medical profession that has given most ground—and not the informed athlete—in the tug-of-war over personal health.

In any event, if a program like Dr. Williams's is the best way of finding your bodyprint, the fitness testing programs aren't far behind. A blood workup is an integral part of the basic examination at such places as Vital, the Aerobics Center (Dallas), the Houstonian Preventive Medicine Center, and most university centers. The difference is that the Institute of Health Research necessarily makes its blood tests at the same time of day and same time of year, every year—and three of them, over a period of several weeks, for added accuracy. They're interested in minute changes, not in comparing you to a national norm. One of the authors of this book had a blood test from a fitness center in the midst of the institute's series, and the results were quite different on two of the twenty-three variables. At present, the fitness centers are more concerned with resting heart rate vs. treadmill rate, body-fat content, oxygen uptake, and strength of handgrip and leg-press. They don't have the expertise to analyze your blood beyond telling you the obvious danger signs. But there's no reason why they can't move in the direction of "health watch" as the news gets around.

Dr. Reginald Cherry, director of the Houston center, is typical of the new breed of "health-watchers." A student of Ken Cooper and the Aerobics Institute, Dr. Cherry naturally emphasizes a complete aerobics program. But he is equally firm in insisting on a diet and lifestyle to support, and not "live off of," the glow of exercise. He pithily describes the "midafternoon crash":

> It is often caused by overcharging the system with carbohydrates, which cause rapid fluctuations in blood-sugar levels and, eventually, a slump. Until your body readjusts to this new level, you live in never-never land.[2]

The carbohydrates he refers to are, of course, not the complex ones in vegetables and fruits, but the simpler ones in alcohol, white flour, and sugar. The "crash" he describes is perhaps the most publicized dietary villain these days, and rightly so. Others refer to it as "sugar shock," "the glucose-insulin trap" (Dr. James T. Cooper), or, technically, "functional hypoglycemia." Dr. Carl Pfeiffer, of the Brain Bio Center, Princeton, New Jersey, has delivered the most recent and telling summation of the case against "the sugar disease," a case that had its beginnings with the research of Dr. Seale Harris in 1922. Now that exercise physiologists are beginning to balance their programs with attention to these basic dietary considerations, they are joining hands with a third major group of testers. They are opening the door to what is known in a cumbersome way as *orthomolecular medicine.*

THE FOOD DOCTORS

In a sense, this book is nothing more than a new way of presenting the basic tenets of what Linus Pauling and other orthomolecularists feel is the "new medicine." It's a medicine based on getting the right nutrients in the body—*for each individual body!* You might assume that this is an obvious and commendable goal. Accordingly, you might assume that the medical world looks kindly on this approach. As we have seen in discussing such a simple thing as the nutritional value of butter, however, the most rational of men resist change. "New medicine"? Ha!

When Linus Pauling delivered a keynote address at the most recent convention of the National Orthomolecular Medical Society (NOMS), a bystander might have felt that he was witnessing an historic turning point in medicine. This patriarch of a scientist—the only person other than Marie Curie to have won two Nobel Prizes—recited the evidence for the orthomolecular approach to preventing and treating disease. He summarized his own case for vitamin C against the common cold and cancer in a masterful presentation of new studies and patient answers to his critics. Then he electrified the room with a most sanguine prediction: In five years, most of the doctors in the country would be practicing this kind of medicine!

Alas, the bystander would not read any of this in a report on the convention in the next day's newspaper. Nor would more than a handful of doctors take kindly to the suggestion that in a few years they would be dispensing zinc tablets, let alone vitamin C pills, for such ailments as arthritis.

Why? Some would see the inevitable capitalistic hand in the background. Dr. Michael Lesser, president of NOMS, recently won a victory for orthomolecular *psychiatry* by receiving approval from the state of California to establish an experimental program in three counties as an alternative to conventional psychiatric treatment. The heads of medical departments at the leading state universities bitterly fought his program. Why, a reporter wanted to know, was there so much opposition to his vitamin-and-mineral form of treatment? Dr. Lesser pointed out that there is no profit potential in unpatentable products, and therefore tremendous economic pressure by the pharmaceutical industry to promote *drugs*.

This oft-repeated fact, nevertheless, fails to account for the well-nigh universal rejection of megavitamin therapy by the medical profession. Perhaps economics is a factor there, too. More understandable, I think, is the general reluctance—on the part of any professional group—to embrace the "fringes" of their field of knowledge.

Anything that lays claim to being a near panacea is suspect. Dr. Pauling and his prestigious colleagues in this field (Irwin Stone, Abram Hoffer, Carl C. Pfeiffer, Harold Rosenberg, to name a few) are well aware of this criticism, and their answer is utterly convincing. We simply are not aware of the pervasiveness of the vitamin C deficiency! (We will come to the vitamin controversy in a later chapter.)

Others, like Dr. George Williams, would grant the preventive properties of orthomolecular treatment, but insist that the curative powers of vitamins and minerals are a long way from clear-cut demonstration. The orthomolecularists, of course, aren't willing to accept half a loaf.

Finally, the diagnostic approach of the "food doctors" seems to put conventional practitioners off. They employ blood tests, of course; but they also take snips of hair from the nape of the neck and analyze them for mineral deficiencies. And they are great advocates of the glucose-tolerance test. Believe it or not, hypoglycemia (the "glucose-insulin trap," "sugar shock," the "midafternoon crash") is still not part of the lexicon of *most doctors*. To them, the glucose-tolerance test is some sort of razzle-dazzle. To quote Lesser or Pfeiffer or Hoffer on the critical nature of this test would prove nothing: they advocate it. Nor are the skeptics convinced by evidence that few medical tests are so well researched, so widely practiced, and so *generally helpful*.

Anyone who seems tagged with an undefinable ailment, who is suspected of mild depression or schizophrenia, or who has serious problems with diet should avail himself or herself of this test.

DOES ANYBODY TALK TO ANYBODY ELSE?

Finally, the people who would like to tell you what your bodyprint is seem to be hopelessly out of touch with each other. No wonder a doctor, who has trouble enough keeping up with two or three medical journals, is unwilling to explore the claims of those who seem to be on the fringe of his profession. There are some extremes that excite the imagination but dismay rational engagement. In his fascinating book, *Mortal Lessons*, Dr. Richard Selzer tells of the Eastern gurus who make a prognostication and a medical history *with apparent accuracy* after a few minutes' examination of one's pulse. There are many specialists who examine the iris—the colored part of the eye—and can tell you more about past and present physical conditions than you could possibly get from a blood test. I know of a biochemist who has helped hundreds of people correct nutritional deficiencies simply by examining their skin, the size and configuration of white spots on their fingernails, the color of their tongues, and so forth. All of this is good, insofar as it's related to rational explanation and not some sort of astrology of the body. The problem is—there seems to be no common ground to pull all these "sciences" together.

At the moment, physicians in orthomolecular medicine have the best chance of making a beachhead in the territory of conventional medicine. The general reader no doubt would prefer to think of them as the "food doctors"—but even healing with food has a bad reputation. Undeservedly. They *are* doctors. They have simply asked a few more questions than were required of them by convention. And there's a curious side effect of this on medical research: they've shown that human subjects cannot be treated as equals in terms of medical health just because they're not visibly sick. Everyone is only *relatively* healthy. Everyone has his or her own health characteristics. So what happens to all the precise studies of human subjects, all the statistical analysis between control groups and study groups, *if the basic assumption of their equality of health is fallacious?* Will all the key studies of modern medicine have to be repeated?

For you, the lesson is clear. All these people are trying to listen to your body. But you—and *only you*—have a ringside seat. In the following chapters we'll see (1) how you can discover a good many facets of your bodyprint by yourself, and (2) how you can use that knowledge to make your old age a *ripe* old age.

FIVE

Conquering the Number-One Killer: Old Age

As a deputy medical examiner for the city of Los Angeles, I studied the causes of death in one of the world's largest metropolitan areas—then with a population center of six million. Since I worked for taxpayers, I felt that they were entitled to know what was killing them. When an electrical hazard killed someone, I sent investigators out to find and correct the hazard. We should learn from our mistakes, so that no one else will get hurt. Safety rules for driving, skin diving, and other stressful activities often result only from tragic accidents. The rules should lessen your chances of the same mishap.

But what about old age? Certainly it is the biggest killer and crippler there is. Or is it?

Yes, if I use my definition of "old age," it *is* the biggest threat we face. It can appear as arthritis, cancer, heart disease, stroke, emphysema, cirrhosis, and a variety of other degenerative conditions. Anything that commonly kills people over forty and rarely kills a teenager might be called old age. In this chapter you'll see why I consider this a good working definition and not just a matter of semantics.

WHO GETS OLD?

The medical examiner often has to determine the age of the deceased, when the identity is uncertain. He becomes very good at estimating biological age; and usually this fits with the actual chronological age. I became interested in the *exceptions*.

Some people die of "old age" in their early years—often under age forty—because their arteries fill up with fatty deposits, or atherosclerosis. Others reach age ninety or one hundred and still have very young-looking arteries—like a teenager's.

One day they brought in a jogger wearing a dark blue sweatsuit. He had been jogging with his back to traffic at dawn. The driver did not see him. Many bones were broken, and he had died at the scene. Since he had no identification, the medical examiner listed him as a "John Doe" with an estimated age of fifty-five. Almost a week went by before an abandoned car was reported belonging to a man about seventy-four. It was about ten miles from the scene where the jogger was hit, and the connection wasn't made right away. Obviously, the medical examiner had underestimated the age because of the absence of atherosclerosis, together with the high level of fitness: a lean, muscular appearance. Relatives identified the jogger. Thus began my suspicion that *aging could be avoided*, for a while at least.

That was many years ago, and since then I have made a study of athletes. *Some age, others do not.*

NOT ALL KINDS OF EXERCISE
PROTECT AGAINST AGING

Sustained aerobic exercise has well-known beneficial effects on the cardiovascular system. The exercise need not be very heavy, but it must be sustained to have that effect; short, violent bursts of exercise don't help. In one study, long-distance runners (aerobic metabolism) were found to have high levels of the protective HDL-cholesterol described earlier, while ice-hockey players (anaerobic metabolism) had normal or low levels.[1]

I have reviewed autopsy slides on middle-distance champions

and other athletes who were very fast or very strong. They did show aging—progression of atherosclerosis—while they were still very fit for their sport!

One cross-country skier trained up to an Olympic level of fitness several times in his late teens and twenties. He was a construction worker, and was always very strong. Although he was a nonsmoker, he died before age thirty-five of atherosclerosis. His arteries showed a very hot, inflammatory reaction to cholesterol—"fast plaque," I call it. He loved charbroiled steaks, and often ate more than one a day. His diet was therefore very low in essential fatty acids and fiber. It contained cholesterol oxide—a toxic lipid oxide from charbroiling. (You will recall that Imai produced injury to arteries in twenty-four hours using cholesterol oxide—see Chapter Three.)

Another middle-distance champion stayed in racing shape all his life and died from atherosclerosis around age forty. He was a nonsmoker. His arteries showed generalized thickening and inflammation without a large amount of cholesterol—the picture I associate with a diet high in *trans*-fat. He was winning races each year, but never finished a marathon. His usual distance for racing was ten kilometers and under—about six miles. Retrospective diet observations showed a pattern of fast foods, low in fiber, low in EFA, and high in *trans*-fat. (Animal experiments have shown that a semipurified, cholesterol-free diet can cause atherosclerosis if *trans*-fat is present.) [2]

These two cases suggested to me that all types of exercise did not offer protection. Aerobic, endurance-type sports appeared to protect, while short, fast, anaerobic sports did not.

HOW OLD ARE YOU, BIOLOGICALLY?

I have looked at autopsies on athletes in terms of their biological age, not their chronological age. Some of the older endurance athletes appeared much younger than "brute" or "spurt" athletes of the same age. In fact, one of the youngest sets of arteries I have ever seen came from a long-distance runner who was over a hundred years of age!

My view is that *your life expectancy is proportional to the distance you can cover on foot!*

I know joggers who get into trouble with leg pains when they try to go beyond their regular two miles a day; and I know marathoners who regularly finish races longer than fifty miles. By anyone's measurement, the fifty-milers will be *younger*, biologically, than the joggers who cannot exceed two miles. Their body fat will be "friendlier" (more EFAs), their oxygen uptake will be higher, their blood-cholesterol levels will be lower, their blood pressures will be lower, etc. Anything you associate with old age should be harder to find in the fifty-milers than the two-milers. Even arthritis!

I think of heart disease and arthritis as signs of old age, even if they appear in your twenties or thirties. Obviously, when you are disabled with arthritis and arteriosclerosis, you are drawing closer to the end of your life span. Fortunately, the process seems to be reversible. I have met a hundred cardiac patients who became marathon runners—running twenty-six-mile marathons after improving their lifestyles. They stopped smoking and changed their exercise and eating habits. Now they are in better shape than when they were teenagers; they think of ten or twenty miles of jogging as an outing of sight-seeing and socializing.

You have control of your biological age through your habits of exercise and eating. As a member of the aerobics generation, you should get biologically younger every year. One way to celebrate is to run your age—a mile for every year. A fifty-year-old who can jog fifty miles in one day is just a teenager, really!

CONSIDER THE ALTERNATIVES: DIETS THAT CAN KILL

Just how hard is it to commit dietary suicide? Not hard. How long will it take?

Wino Diet

When I first joined the medical examiner's office, I examined the body of a man in his early thirties. He had arrived in California only three months earlier. He didn't find a job, so he lived in his parked car, drinking large amounts of inexpensive table wine. I estimated from his liver that the alcohol molecule had supplied over 60 percent of his calories on most days. His liver had quickly enlarged and filled with fat. Death was caused by pneumonia. (All of our defenses against infections rely upon an adequate supply of proteins from the liver; without a good liver, the nearest germ can quickly kill you.)

Trans-Fat Diet

Hydrogenated vegetable oils, starch, and sugar make up the bulk of the calories in semisynthetic fast foods. I have seen sections of arteries from a nonsmoker around forty years old, who exercised regularly but died of atherosclerosis. The arteries contained *trans*-fat, and his diet was highly refined. I estimated from his arteries that refined calories accounted for over 40 percent of his diet. It was low in fiber and EFAs.

As we have seen, hydrogenated peanut oil caused atherosclerosis in monkeys in five months, and hydrogenated coconut oil and sucrose caused atherosclerosis in rabbits in ten months.[3]

Both of these diets are available in supermarkets: solid peanut butter is hydrogenated; and cream "substitutes" for coffee usually contain hydrogenated coconut oil.

Sugar Diet

Sucrose is often disguised on a label by a variety of other names. Some nutritionists suggest that manufacturers use a variety of sugars so that no single one will have to be listed first in the list of ingredients—as is required by law if it is the major ingredient.

Rabbits developed atherosclerosis in less than a year with a diet that was 63 percent sucrose. This diet was low in fat and free of cholesterol.[4]

Heavy sugar intake is possible from a wide variety of foods:
Fruits: jams, jellies, canned fruit with thick syrup
Dairy: flavored yogurts, ice cream
Bakery: pastries, cakes, cookies

Cereals: packaged breakfast foods

Meats: candied ham

Vegetables: candied yams, many canned vegetables

Snacks: Almost all semisynthetic snacks have added sugars. The soft drinks, candy bars, and cupcake-like objects may be little more than sugar, coloring, flavoring, and stabilizers.

Caffeine and Tobacco Diet

By exceeding fifteen cups of coffee a day and three packs of cigarettes, cardiac disease can be brought on before age thirty. The high concentrations of nicotine, caffeine, and carbon monoxide can damage arteries without a high-fat diet. By using instant coffee, the caffeine intake can be raised to very dangerous levels with ease. If the tobacco is smoked indoors with windows closed, the effect is multiplied by the breathing of secondhand smoke from room air. I have seen several deaths from this combination. Oddly enough, friends and relatives of the deceased usually think nothing of coffee and cigarettes for "breakfast" and "coffee breaks" throughout the day!

Combination Diet for Premature Death

By far the most common suicide diet includes all of the above: a little wine plus margarines and shortenings plus sugary treats plus caffeine and nicotine. When these dangerous calories exceed 40 percent of your intake—and *that* is *very* easy to do— then the arteries start to age rapidly.

I find that a suicide diet is usually a subconscious act resulting from depression. Look at the mood elevators in each part of the diet: alcohol, sugar, artificial flavors, nicotine and caffeine— *all* capable of inducing transient stimulation. When I ask a patient why his shopping cart contains such items, he uses all the social excuses. The wino drinks to be happy; the fast-food eater is rushed and has no time to invest in his diet; the sugar-eater wants an energy lift; the caffeine and nicotine users are addicted to their molecules. They all find happiness by putting the wrong things into their mouths.

And that sort of "happiness" can kill—or at least age one significantly.

INTIMATIONS OF IMMORTALITY

The fact that we *look* older every year leads us to assume that our vital organs are also aging at the same rate. Not so. We can speak realistically of the "absence of aging." If you look like a teenager on the autopsy table, you are a success. I have seen sections of arteries from joggers from seventy to one hundred ten years old that looked as if they were from teenagers. The causes of death were the same as in a teenage population— accidents, homicide, suicide, infections, tumors, and a few other rare conditions.

If I Don't Age, What Will I Die Of?
Old age kills only two thirds of the adults between 40 and 70. If you can stop aging, you still must worry about the other third, things that can kill teenagers. If the death rate drops to one third, then you can stretch out the 40–70 age range sixty years to 40–130. The teenage causes will still be there. My goal is to make sure that everyone remains a teenager until he or she dies from some rare accident. Then, without "old age" there is no need for anyone to retire to a rest home. You can retire from one job, go to school again, and learn a new skill. While you are at school, you can join the track team and enter age-group competition.

What Kind of Diet Prevents Aging?
Whatever helps you run beyond the eighteen-mile mark. Getting to the twenty-six-mile mark in the marathon requires adequate silicon, vitamin C, and EFAs—all associated with protection against aging.

What Kind of Exercise Prevents Aging?
Slow activities which require endurance beyond the eighteen-mile mark. Being able to *walk* or jog twenty-six miles is the key. Speed and strength play no role, and may actually do harm if they cause increased injuries.

What If I Don't Know Anything about Diet Chemistry?

Just follow your instincts. If it helps you cover greater distances on foot, then it is good for you. If something makes you feel that you cannot run or walk better, then stop eating it. Your body will quickly sort out your diet, improving it.

What If I Can't Run My Age?

Then run a mile farther each year; that makes you "younger" than the year before, since the *distance covered on foot* keeps going up.

How Fast Do I Have to Go?

There is no qualifying speed. A mile is about a hundred calories, no matter how fast or slow you cover the distance. Walking counts. There are pleasant social twenty-four-hour events in several places around the world; more are on the way. If you wanted to saunter along with the crowd at a twenty-minute-mile pace—three miles per hour—you could do thirty miles in ten hours, nap four hours, and do another thirty miles in the last ten hours for a total of sixty miles in twenty-four hours! More about this in Chapter Ten.

What If My Distance Gets Shorter?

Then you're living wrong! Check your diet and other living habits. Talk with joggers your own age to see what they think is helping them improve their distance. If you slow your pace enough, you should always be able to increase the distance. Calories can be replaced every mile—soup, beer, fruit and vegetable juices, soft drinks, and even the light meals of carbohydrates like pasta. A nap now and then helps too. A day is a long time, but once you get out beyond sixty miles you may want to extend it to a two-day run. Make your own rules to fit your body's needs.

Will Exercise Help Menopausal Depression?

Menopausal depression can be linked with the withdrawal of the sex hormone in both males and females. Vigorous exercise, started at least nine months before menopause, can create a bigger demand for this same type of hormone—a steroid hormone from the adrenal gland—and thus protect you when the sex organ (ovary or testis) stops making as much sex hormone. Apparently, primitive man developed his muscles and his adrenal gland enough to carry him through menopause without depression. However, urban man is weak and soft, has small adrenal glands, and depends on his gonads for steroids. When the gonads cut back at menopause, there is not enough adrenal function to keep the mood elevated.

X rays of the spine are a good way to document the level of steroid hormone activity. Inactive women lose bone calcium from the spine at menopause, and the aorta gains calcium; but active women do not! (*Active* means jogging six miles three times a week.)

LET YOUR EXERCISE TALK TO YOU!

Both of the vigorous athletes I mentioned before, the skier and the middle-distance runner, had diets that contained dangerous types of fat: cholesterol oxide for the skier and *trans*-fat for the runner. So, I began to suspect that exercise, itself, did not protect against aging. Smoking, exercise, and diet all play a role. However, because of the demands of the sport, the marathon runners appear to be protected, since they usually do not smoke and they avoid the types of fats that they cannot use for energy (the toxic lipid oxides, *trans*-fat, grease, and saturated fats).

Diet is dictated by the sport, and the diet also dictates performance in the sport. The two go together.

The Five Ways to Increase the Magic HDL

The high-density lipoproteins (HDLs) are the lipids or fats with a lot of good protein mixed in; more protein means that the molecule is heavier, thus the "high-density." Your good cholesterol travels around in your blood with a lot of protein and is called HDL-cholesterol. If it is really high, say over 55 mg/dl, then you are in a group where atherosclerosis is very rare.

There are several ways to raise your protective HDL levels:

1. lose weight;
2. increase exercise;
3. increase intake of vitamin C;
4. increase beer intake; and
5. add a whole egg to your diet.

You can lower your HDL and increase your risk by doing the opposite, plus smoking and eating refined foods. Thus, your HDL will drop if you stop exercising, gain weight, stop drinking beer, stop taking vitamin C, and switch from whole eggs to powdered egg or artificial egg. As your HDL drops, your risk increases! And you have seven ways to lose HDL, only five to gain it.

How an "Experiment of One" Taught Us about Vitamin C and HDL

One of my running buddies, a man in his early seventies, was once a heavy smoker. About ten years ago he stopped smoking and went on a vigorous walking program. He had never exercised before, but his bad habits had finally caught up to him. At age sixty-two he was disabled by anginal chest pain. His doctor told him he flunked his exercise test, and an angiogram showed that all his coronary arteries were closed. The surgeons did not like the looks of his arteries. They looked beaded, with many narrowed areas in a row. There was no good place to put in a coronary bypass.

Little was known about the use of exercise and vitamin C for coronary heart disease ten years ago. But he really had no choice. The surgeons would not operate, so he had to stop smoking and go on an exercise program. He also read a great deal, coming across the reports on possible benefits from vitamin C. He took over a gram each day. It raised his cholesterol level, and he felt better. He thought that the raised cholesterol meant that vitamin C was removing bad cholesterol from his arteries! (Nothing was known about the effect of vitamin C in raising the protective HDL-cholesterol back in those days.)

Luck was on his side, and he gradually worked up to walking in twenty-six-mile marathons. He jogs a little and walks a little. He still sees cardiologist-coaches, but he looks like any other runner on the roads, wearing bright jogging clothes, drinking beer, and wearing official entry numbers in races.

His original coronary angiogram showed "four-vessel disease," reported as 100, 90, 90, and 95 percent narrowing—about the most severe disease I have seen in a cardiac athlete. He taught us a lot about the potential for rehabilitation that a dedicated patient has. And he taught me a lot about the value of adequate vitamin C intake!

How Smoking Ages You

Middle-aged men and women will have three toes in their crow's feet—those little wrinkles in the outer corners of their eyes. These "smile wrinkles" are normal. About one more toe is added for each twenty years. However, 350 pack of cigarettes (a pack a day for a year, or a pack-year) also adds another toe. Dermatologists often take high-contrast black-and-white profile photographs and bring them to conventions where other dermatologists estimate the pack-years each patient has smoked. The accuracy of this crow's-foot counting is striking! Anyone can do it—just count the lines and subtract three to get the number of pack-years smoked.

The reason for the lines is obvious once you look at skin samples under the microscope. The oxides in the smoke accelerate tissue aging; and the tissue *looks older!* Oxides destroy vitamins C and E and expose the fats to oxidation. When the antioxidants go, so do the fibers that hold the tissue together—elastic fibers that allow the skin to stretch and bounce back intact.

By the same process, smoking cancels out the benefits of even a good diet. The oxides in the smoke destroy vitamins C and E. That leaves the EFAs exposed to oxidation, forming toxic lipid oxides. Since the EFAs are needed for fuel in endurance exercise, few smokers can run beyond the six-mile mark. (The first six miles can be run on stored glycogen, a carbohydrate.)

Since vitamin C is needed to form strong cartilage in the knees and strong collagen in tendons, the smoker will get into problems with knee and tendon pains because of his lower vitamin C levels—another reason why few smokers can run far. "Smoker's knee" is simply a painful swollen knee in a smoker who has low levels of vitamin C.

Smoking decreases the amount of oxygen your blood can carry because carbon monoxide combines with hemoglobin, blocking oxygen uptake.

Smoking increases the risk of sudden death during exercise because the heart muscle becomes irritable and has a tendency to beat irregularly during anaerobic, stressful activity. Even a good exercise test from a good cardiologist doesn't tell a smoker when he can expect trouble with his heart rhythm. It's too unpredictable.

It's doubtful that adding vitamins C and E to the diet will cancel out the effects of *current* smoking. However, once smoking is stopped, the future aging of the skin and tendons can be slowed by raising tissue levels of these antioxidants. The parallel-aging theory states that your skin and your aorta "age" together. Therefore, those with "old" skin can get into trouble with atherosclerosis earlier!

Lung cancer is always a threat after 7,000 packs of cigarettes have been smoked (about a pack a day for twenty years). The dose of carcinogens in the tobacco smoke is large enough to produce a tumor. However, if you stop smoking after 7,000 packs, the risk of a tumor will *decrease* after about three years, and after six years it will be only about twice that of a non-smoker. Former smokers will never be as low-risk as those who never smoked because there is always some residual damage from the carcinogens in tobacco tar.

However, antioxidants have been shown to decrease the risk of carcinogens in animal work. Again, vitamins C and E were used. Therefore, the former smoker can reduce his residual risk by keeping his tissues saturated with antioxidants.

How the "Lipid Oxide Equation" Tells You When Smoking Is Harmful to You—and Can Help You Stop Smoking!

If you have been able to stop smoking for six weeks in the past, but then started again, you might be interested in this diet trick that makes it easier to stay away from cigarettes. *Eat more foods rich in EFAs and vitamin E when you are not smoking.* This will raise the level of polyunsaturates in the fat. When it is high enough (after about six weeks) the smoke will be very irritating because it will actually react with your tissues, forming toxic lipid oxides. *You will not enjoy smoking because of the irritation,* and can continue not smoking. Unfortunately, or fortunately, you will not enjoy smoky rooms and so will stop seeing friends who smoke. This is simply a chemical reaction: smoke + lipids = toxic lipid oxides.

How Your Achilles Tendon Tells You about
Your Protection against Heart Disease

One reason why marathon runners appear to be immune to atherosclerosis is that they have tough Achilles tendons, and human-autopsy studies have shown that *the coronary arteries and Achilles tendons have parallel aging.* Old tendons go with old arteries. And, conversely, a young tendon means that you have young arteries.[5]

If you can walk the twenty-six-mile marathon distance, then you must have a pretty tough tendon—and, if the theory is correct, all the tissues in the body will be young.

What keeps tissues young?

Many things, but among them are clearly the food-fiber factor (silicon) and the antioxidants (vitamins C and E). Of course, you have to have a healthy liver and adequate protein in the diet to make good tendons and arteries, and you have to avoid oxidants that might destroy vitamin C. But all these things should be taken care of in the Whole Life Diet.

The Clearest Message of All: Your Cravings for
Food after a Race or Walk

Marathoners need more EFAs than do other sportsmen, because they burn more. Therefore, they crave more, eat more, and have more EFAs in their tissues. We know from human-autopsy studies that a high level of EFAs in tissue is associated with lower numbers of heart-attack deaths. It appears that the marathoners' fuel may contribute significant protection against atherosclerosis.

The beer they drink may also protect them. Beer, alone, has been known to raise the level of protective HDL-cholesterol, and lower the incidence of fatal atherosclerosis. Beer contains silicon. Silicon, by itself, is associated with less atherosclerosis. Now you can see the pattern of food cravings we discused in Chapter Two. But, remember, we're talking about "associations," not cause and effect.

Many Joggers, Including Marathoners, Have Died While
Running. Why Didn't EFAs and Silicon Protect Them?

Autopsies have shown two types of death in joggers. Those with progressive atherosclerosis will have myocardial infarction or coronary thrombosis—something recent in the heart to explain death. In some cases there is death of single muscle fibers, a microscopic infarction, and the death is caused by arrhythmia—an irregular heartbeat. But there had to be a preexisting condition, which should have been known.

The other type of death is *not* due to atherosclerosis. These deaths are rare, but should be carefully studied, because these conditions can kill teenagers too. Some examples:

A virus can settle in the heart muscle and cause the fatal arrhythmia at rest or during exercise.

Caffeine or other stimulants can be dangerous if used during vigorous exercise on a hot day. Usually these deaths caused by stimulants have been during races, not jogging.

Exertion-induced heat illness can be seen in races as short as six miles. In severe cases there can be kidney damage, brain death, or myocardial infarction. This is what is behind George Sheehan's maxim: "Heat is the only thing that can kill the healthy athlete."

After the "jogging death" is correctly classified, then safety rules can be applied. Common sense will tell you to avoid dehydration, heat, stimulants, and carbon monoxide. However, if your heart is suspected of being abnormal, then you also should have a treadmill test so you can exercise at a safe level. See Chapter Four for "fitness" testing.

Once you have finished a twenty-six-mile marathon, I consider you protected from atherosclerosis; but that doesn't mean that you can't die from other things. Remember, I consider marathon runners to be "teenagers" because I have studied *autopsies* on many of them. *Something* has been killing them! Your job is to keep an eye open for the things that can kill you, and avoid them. What is sad to see is an otherwise intelligent person avoid aerobic exercise on the pretext that "joggers die every day."

Is Food Fiber a Cure-All?

To read about all the things it can protect you from, you might think of it as that. However, some fiber works better than others. How do you know you are getting the right kind of fiber? Watch your stools. If they are 25 cm long (about 10 inches) and if they float, then fiber intake is probably adequate. Also, the active ingredient, silicon, helps hold your joints and tendons together; for this reason, the distance you can cover on foot is an index of your fiber intake.

Some of the conditions associated with *low fiber* include gallstones, varicose veins, hemorrhoids, cancer and other diseases of the colon, and atherosclerosis leading to heart attack and stroke. Adding fiber to a refined diet may not change this; you have to go back to the original foods and eat them whole with their original fiber.

Diabetes is easier to manage on a full-fiber diet and a vigorous exercise program.

Arthritis also responds to a full-fiber diet, probably because of the higher intake of silicon.

When Is It Too Late to Start?

We know only that some patients have had far-advanced disease and then succeeded in reaching a high level of fitness. One man with an artificial heart valve has run a marathon. Many with myocardial infarction and bypass surgery have run marathons and longer races, up to sixty-two miles (100 km). The total number of cardiac athletes is only about 150 at the marathon distance, but several hundred have reached the six-mile goal and are doing fine, so far. The slowest marathoner in a recent run we had wasn't a cardiac patient. He took ten hours to cover the twenty-six miles, so if you are slower than that you will just set a new record for slowness! There is no time limit! It's never too late to start aerobic exercise. It's too late when you stop.

What If I Have Liver Disease?

Liver disease is usually caused by alcohol abuse, an addiction that can be switched to a running addiction. The minimum dose for the switch seems to be twenty-one hours—over a month or two—of slow jogging at 70 percent effort with a group of five to seven joggers. The patients who were put in this program had a cardiologist-coach to tell them what was safe. They jogged and walked for an hour, three times a week, with their group. They had to go slow, because competition would block the addiction process. After six weeks on the program, they were able to stop drinking, but they *had* to continue jogging an hour almost every day because now they were addicted to running instead. Also, as in any addiction, they had to keep increasing the dose of mileage! In the early stages, they were satisfied with a few miles. Each month another mile was "needed." By the end of the first year, they were running half-marathons, or thirteen miles. After two years, they were doing marathons and longer races.

How Do I Know If My Liver Is Damaged?

The liver handles amino acids to make proteins. When there is severe damage I can see changes in blood proteins. Even the red blood cells look unusual—they're larger and paler than normal. If you can jog your six miles, three times a week, and your knees don't hurt, then the liver is strong enough to handle the protein you need to keep your knee cartilage together. If you have been in the hospital with liver damage and now are running six miles, then the damage isn't severe enough to worry about. *It takes a pretty good liver to hold the knee together.* Heavy drinkers can get pain—"drinker's knee"—as a warning that their diet is a mess. As I keep saying, one of the best reasons to jog is to keep tabs on the nutrients in the diet.

In the blood tests mentioned in Chapter Four, an enzyme known as gamma glutyl transpeptidase (GGTP) is an indicator in the liver cells of increased alcohol consumption. But the "drinker's-knee test" seems quite valid to me.

What If I Already Have Emphysema?

Emphysema, or "smoker's lung," is related to the total dose of cigarettes smoked in a lifetime. At autopsy, you can almost guess the number of pack-years the patient smoked just by looking at the lung damage with the naked eye. One pack a day for twenty years is called "twenty pack-years." It takes about twenty pack-years before consistent, measurable damage shows up that will interfere with an exercise program. However, the damage will not progress if you stop smoking and start jogging. (Unfortunately, the risk of lung cancer remains higher than for a nonsmoker for several years. The cancer-causing tars may have already damaged some cells in the lung, so there is a period after you stop smoking during which a tumor could still show up. However, once you have stopped for six years, the risk is about the same as for a nonsmoker.)

Emphysema responds rather dramatically to a vigorous exercise program. Perhaps diet plays a role in this. Animal studies do show that the antioxidants protect against lung damage from tobacco smoke. It is logical to think that human lung tissue benefits from the higher intake of vitamins C and E that is associated with vigorous exercise.

What If I Take Medication for Arthritis?

Patients reduced their arthritis medication when they were on a high-fiber diet and a vigorous exercise program. Silicon and vitamin C may help reduce the need for arthritis pain killers. I think that mileage can be substituted for medication in most cases. Our joints are designed to be used. Rest only allows the bones to grow soft. If a joint is immobilized too long it will grow stiff. You must stay active!

Even Rheumatoid Arthritis Seems to Be Treatable with Diet. Is It the Linoleic Acid?

McCormick and associates reported that a naturally occurring mixture of essential fatty acids, *naudicelle*, did suppress antibody production in tissue culture. They grew lymphocytes in culture and stimulated them to make antibodies. However, they were able to suppress the amount of antibody produced by adding naudicelle. Now they are trying it on patients with rheumatoid arthritis. Some patients already claim to be improved after three months.

The theory is this: Rheumatoid arthritis is a painful disease of joints due to abnormal antibodies being formed, which attack the joint membrane. Your body makes a mistake and uses the weapons that are supposed to fight infections, but they attack the joints instead. Treatments that suppress antibody production, such as the use of cortisone, have helped these patients in the past; however, cortisone is too dangerous for regular use. Hence, the search for a natural food item that will do the same thing, ideally without side effects.[6]

I have seen reports that a vigorous exercise program did help some patients with rheumatoid arthritis. A possible explanation could be the increased intake of vitamin E and linoleic acid. The naudicelle is 70 percent linoleic acid! Perhaps the exercising patients were already getting their EFAs someplace else, and this helped reduce their rheumatoid-arthritis symptoms. Also, the intake of vitamin C, silicon, and other nutrients could have improved local joint conditions. Notice our familiar trio of vitamin C, EFAs, and silicon again!

So we see that the major "killer" diseases of our age can very well be thought of as one disease—the lack of the nutrients of a *young* body. This is why I think of aging itself as the real killer. The hue and cry today, of course, is about heart disease. And it is the *immediate* cause of more deaths in people in the "prime of life" than cancer or the other diseases mentioned above. Let's look at atherosclerosis, therefore, in more detail.

SIX

Food for Your Heart

When Karl von Rokitansky, one of the early giants of pathology, wrote his textbook back in 1852, he thought that arteries filled up with atherosclerotic fat in much the same way that pipes fill with calcium scale.[1] He thought that small blood clots encrusted the inner walls of arteries, thickening them and narrowing the openings. Recently, this encrustation theory has been expanded to include the loss of the pavement-like lining cells inside the arteries. Without these cells, the inner walls of the arteries would be rough and attract small clots.[2]

I see two dietary factors playing a role in this theory. First, the clotting of blood is controlled by small blood particles called platelets, which are rich in fat. Marathon runners eat a lot of "friendly" fat (EFAs) and probably have "friendly" platelets that would not cause abnormal clots. Second, the pavement-lining cells inside the artery are held in place by cement, which depends on high vitamin C levels. The marathon runner eats foods rich in vitamin C to protect his tendons and, at the same time, to protect the lining cells of his arteries so clots won't stick to them.

Rudolf Virchow was more impressed with the fat in the wall of the artery. In 1856, he suggested that the arterial wall thickened because fats entered the wall from the blood.[3] In some cases, the fat was inside cells and the numbers of cells increased; in other cases, the fat was outside of cells and formed pools that grew.

Again, I can see a dietary explanation. Fat certainly can enter the arteries from the blood; but it gets into the blood through our gut. If we eat ten or twenty times more fat than we need, it will just be stored everywhere—in the arteries, but also in the skin, muscles, and other places, giving us a heavy, round body. Too many calories of any kind are dangerous! But then people also can have atherosclerosis. The fat can go into the arterial wall if the wall is made of poor-quality material. Schwarz has suggested that a low-fiber diet leaves our arterial wall deficient in silicon. Fats can accumulate in a low-silicon artery. Also, "unfriendly" fats can attack a normal artery and cause disease. If the fat is inside the cells, causing proliferation, I think of them as *trans*-fats from hydrogenated vegetable oils, but if the fat is outside the cells, forming soft pools of fat in the walls of arteries, then I think of them as grease or toxic lipid oxides from fried foods or charbroiled steaks.

Both Rokitansky and Virchow were partially right, back in the 1850s, more than a hundred years ago. There are several dietary mistakes we can make: too little vitamin C, too little "friendly" fat (EFAs), too little food fiber (silicon) or too much unfriendly fat (hydrogenated oils or burned animal fats). Any one of these mistakes can result in atherosclerosis.

Animals have been used to show that diet causes atherosclerosis. In 1913, Anitschkow fed cholesterol to rabbits and raised their blood-cholesterol levels to ten and twenty times normal.[4] Atherosclerosis-like areas were seen in two months. These diets were very high in fat, far in excess to what rabbits normally eat. Also, the diets were low in fiber, EFAs, and vitamin C. The diets contained toxic lipid oxides also; so the hazard of a pure cholesterol molecule was not shown. Anitschkow only

showed that the disease could be caused by a diet that was
highly abnormal for the rabbit. I agree!

WHAT WE KNOW ABOUT CHOLES-
TEROL FROM HUMAN STUDIES

I'm going to repeat things about butter and eggs and margarine
I've mentioned already. But I think it's important to make a full
and unequivocal case if you're going to trust me enough to stop
worrying about butter and the egg!

I do get a little nervous when I read of massive dietary
studies using hundreds of humans for experimental subjects; but
such studies had to be done. I have mixed feelings for the
medical scientists who devoted decades of their lives to this
work; and, of course, I wish the human subjects did not have to
be used in such studies. But the work has been done; and the
results are published in great detail for all of us to read—and
benefit from.

The Finnish Mental Hospital Study (1959–71) showed no
significant change in total mortality when dairy fats were replaced by vegetable oils; however, there were fewer deaths from
coronary heart disease while vegetable oils were eaten. Fat tissues were biopsied to show that linoleic acid levels rose from
about 10 percent to 30 percent while vegetable oils were eaten.
This resulted in a 50 percent drop in the deaths from heart
attack. There was no other change in lifestyle; smoking and exercise stayed about the same—as did the rest of the diet. The
linoleic-acid levels in the diet were elevated by replacing the
cream in milk with soybean oil, and using a special polyunsaturated margarine instead of butter.[5]

My only criticism of using this study to promote the use of
margarine over butter is that the group on the dairy-fat diet
were also eating "common margarine" with *trans*-fat! The group
on the special polyunsaturated margarine may have been protected, not because they avoided butter, but because they
avoided common margarine—the hydrogenated vegetable oil I
am afraid of! Before we use this study to encourage the use of

vegetable instead of animal fats, we should also remember that no significant change in the *total* death rate was seen.[6]

Soybean oil did lower total cholesterol by 15 percent, but there was no discussion of protective HDL-cholesterol back in those years. Also, the *trans*-fat and lipid-oxide content of the diets were not known. Therefore, I looked at a more recent study at a V.A. hospital in the United States.[7]

I have commented upon this study before.[8] The 424 subjects ate margarine, skim milk, and imitation ice cream, while the "controls" ate butter and eggs. They were followed for eight years and there was no difference in the *total* death rate of the two groups. Also, meticulous autopsy studies showed no difference in the degree of atherosclerosis in each group. However, there were fewer heart attacks and more tumors in the group on margarine. The number of heart attacks was almost exactly the same as the number of heavy smokers (*heavy* smokers used over a pack a day) in each group!

The butter-eaters had 70 heavy smokers; there were 70 deaths from coronary heart disease! The margarine-users included only 45 heavy smokers, and they had only 48 coronary deaths!

The total death rate in both groups was about the same (283 subjects on polyunsaturates died; 279 controls died).

The cancer deaths (20 butter-eaters; 33 margarine-eaters) did suggest that the polyunsaturates might be hazardous to your health; but when multiple trials are combined, this carcinogenic effect was not significant.[9]

However, I continue to worry about extracted oils, whether they are saturated or polyunsaturated. Extracted oils are too "processed" to suit me; since they lack protein, vitamins, and silicon, they can be eaten in excess. Remember, a polyunsaturated diet shortened the mean life span of mice.[10]

Therefore, I concluded from this eight-year study that *smoking* causes heart attacks, and polyunsaturates may be hazardous in the extracted, semisynthetic form of margarine.

Dr. Morris of London tried to show a relationship between diet and heart disease with a meticulous survey of free-living humans.[11] He found that men with fewer heart attacks ate more calories (and exercised more), and they ate more cereal fiber (obtaining the protective element silicon).

Hugh Sinclair, also an English physician, looked over the same information and concluded that it was not the cereal fiber at all but another group of protective elements in whole-wheat flour. Sinclair thinks that the fewer heart attacks were due to a higher intake of "essential fatty acids (EFAs), vitamin B_6, which is closely related to them, and vitamin E, which powerfully protects them." [12]

Both Sinclair and Morris see the hazards of bleached white flour. They have aimed their research and medical pressure on the government policies that affect diet in England. Twenty years ago, Sinclair warned of the public-health hazard of switching from real whole wheat to a partially fortified white flour.[13] Both Sinclair and Morris find that refining wheat is a health hazard, although they differ slightly on the key protective factor. I agree that all of the factors probably play a role—silicon, EFAs, vitamins B_6 and E, plus many other natural elements in the wheat germ and bran. Nothing can be removed without some risk! Evolution has molded our genes to eat grains whole, with all the nutrients. Civilization cannot change that.

The survey by Morris also covered the ratio of polyunsaturates to saturated fats and found no significant difference. There were fewer coronary patients in those with a higher intake of the polyunsaturates, but not few enough to be statistically significant. I think future studies will show that *trans*-fats are dangerous and should not be counted among the polyunsaturates, since they are worse, biologically, than the saturated fats. Such surveys should cover EFAs, silicon, and toxic lipid oxides also. Then we will see significant results! This Morris survey covered 337 men for twenty years, more than adequate time to evaluate a diet had they had the laboratory methods of today.

Is Coffee Unsafe? Or Does It Just Keep Bad Company?

Population studies suggest an *association* between regular coffee-drinking and increased risk of heart attack,[14] but I can think of several explanations for this even if the coffee bean is completely innocent.

Hydrogenated coconut oil and sucrose: This combination was used to induce atherosclerosis in animals in the absence of cholesterol. Some coffee drinkers will not use cream because of their fear of dairy fat (a fear I suspect is unfounded). To whiten their coffee they use a cream substitute, which may contain hydrogenated coconut oil. Add table sugar (sucrose) and you have a combination that is dangerous by itself; no need to worry about the coffee in that cup!

Soft water: Low-silicon soft water caused increased numbers of heart attacks in Finland. If coffee is regularly made with pure soft water (and the rest of your diet is low fiber), you will not have silicon to protect you from heart attack. No need to worry about the coffee in the cup if the water is soft.

Coffee and cigarettes: In this familiar combination, the coffee is not the hazard; the cigarettes are!

Coffee and doughnuts: Here, the doughnut can be the most dangerous, since more hydrogenated vegetable oil can be hidden there, masked by sugars, artificial flavors, and starch.

Even if the coffee bean is innocent, its use is *associated* with other things that are guilty of causing increased heart attack. Even beer, with its higher silicon levels, is a healthier drink than coffee made with soft water. Herbal tea may have high silicon levels if alfalfa, rice straw, or other plant fiber is used. Tea is less likely to be used with artificial whitener. Tea is not as closely associated with cigarettes, either.

Caffeine can be dangerous when excessive intake is combined with vigorous exercise and underlying heart disease; but there are many sources of caffeine other than coffee. Colas are the most prominent. Some tips: green tea (as well as herb teas) are caffeine free; decaffeinated coffees are virtually caffeine free, but expensive; Nescafé is one of the few regular coffees that are about 90 percent caffeine free.

Is the Egg Dangerous?
Why would anyone ask such a question? Where is there evidence that eggs might be dangerous?

Cholesterol is present in eggs, of course, but so is a *complete* list of vitamins, minerals, and amino acids. I have *faith* in the egg because I have seen many of them turn into living baby chicks; all I did was set them under a hen! The egg is alive; and Bassler's first rule is: You can eat anything that's alive!

Who said the egg is dangerous?

Egg *yolks* have been used to produce atherosclerosis in adult monkeys but the monkeys ate a semipurified diet in which egg-yolk fat made up 40 percent of the total calories! [15] This study is not relevant to humans using whole eggs, since the high-quality protein in the egg white is needed to "carry" the cholesterol. The essential amino acids in the egg white must be consumed as part of an optimum diet.[16]

The egg-yolk diet for the monkeys was deficient in fiber, essential fatty acids, and essential amino acids. *Any* refined calorie can cause trouble in such a diet. If your diet is balanced already, the addition of a single egg each day will not cause a lasting rise in the serum cholesterol when compared to the same diet with no egg per day.[17] Furthermore, I believe that the protective HDL-cholesterol can be raised by adding the egg. This is suggested by the charts in the paper by Franzini and Schivi.[18] And, certainly for the aerobics generation, those getting an hour or so of endurance exercise each day, a simple rule for minimum egg intake should be: one egg for each six miles.

In one important study, *diet* cholesterol and *serum* (blood) cholesterol were not related over a wide range of intake.[19] This study used radioactive tracers to prove that diet cholesterol was absorbed, but blood levels were not related to the amount absorbed. So one egg, more or less, is OK.

You will continue to hear reports that egg intake is *associated* with a high blood cholesterol. This is probably true. Most Americans have a couple eggs for breakfast, along with toast, bacon, jelly, coffee, and perhaps a cigarette. Obviously, the egg is the least of the problem in smokers. Also, *grease* has been shown to be more dangerous than egg yolks in Kummerow's experiments on pigs; so the bacon is suspect. The bread is not that safe either, if there are *hydrogenated* oils in the shortening and margarine.

So, the egg is innocent; it has just been keeping bad company—grease and hydrogenated vegetable oils.

The safest way to eat an egg is poached on a baked potato. That way you don't have to worry about the toast with its empty calories of white flour and *trans*-fat in the shortening and margarine. Poached eggs on a baked potato can include ample butter without raising the blood cholesterol if plenty of raw onions are added. Onions cancel out the cholesterol in butter and a butter-and-onion meal actually *lowered* the blood cholesterols in humans! [20]

What Is the Story behind Raw Eggs?

Many athletes have tried raw eggs at one time or another, and there is considerable folklore suggesting that this form of protein is capable of adding extra strength during a heavy training season. I have tried this, myself: raw eggs in beer; raw eggs in various "nogs" with whole milk, fruit, wheat germ, and other secret ingredients. I will encourage any athlete who experiments with "super drinks" using natural ingredients. Since these drinks are raw, it is almost impossible to get a bad molecule into them without spoiling the flavor. Rancid wheat germ, for example, will taste terrible in a nog. So will decaying fruit. Eating something raw almost guarantees that you are getting high-quality protein. So the raw-egg eaters may have something; certainly our Stone Age ancestors did not bother to cook their eggs!

YOU CAN'T EAT CONSPIRACIES . . .

Why should you believe Tom Bassler about cholesterol and eggs rather than the American Heart Association, the Center for Science in the Public Interest, and researchers such as Dr. Mark Hegsted at the Harvard School of Public Health, Dr. A. M. Kligman at the University of Pennsylvania, and many others whose work is the basis for the current official position? Perhaps the best-known nutritionist in America, Dr. Jean Mayer, formerly of Harvard and now president of Tufts College, writes in a syndicated newspaper column:

Although there is some adjustment of cholesterol production in relation to cholesterol intake, the fact is this correction is far less than complete. The consumption of large amounts of dietary cholesterol still increases blood cholesterol.[21]

There are at least three levels on which one can argue for or against such a large proposition as the one that not eating eggs is a protection against heart attacks. One level is the purely scientific: the studies, the laboratory and epidemiological evidence. Another level is the theoretical: reasoning from our knowledge of food and man in general. A third is what might be called the conspiratorial: what economic or other interests are pushing for or against eggs?

I find the last to be the most annoying level of discussion. The reasoning is akin to the *argumentum ad hominem* of the sophist: let's find out who's behind the other side and tear him apart. And the trouble is that this type of argument clouds the other two.

In Chapter One I mentioned the fact that corporations behind vegetable-oil and margarine production obviously have much to gain from the cholesterol scare. But I don't mean to offer corporate greed as an argument against the products they're pushing. (An objective person must always be ready to admit that the opposition may eventually be shown to have been right!) For the same reason I hope that the egg industry isn't pictured as lurking in the background of any study favoring eggs. An article in CSPI's newsletter in late 1978 concluded with these words:

> Whether the egg industry will be able to convince the public that eggs do not influence heart disease remains to be seen. But the egg industry is already counting its chickens.[22]

That same issue raised objections to two of the studies I've cited above in support of eggs.[23] That's fair enough: proper control of experiments is an important scientific issue. But in my opinion any shortcomings in those studies have been more than made up for by the preponderance of supporting evidence of recent years, including early 1979. In his book, *Supernutrition,* gerontologist Richard A. Passwater summarized the evidence tellingly—all the relevant material up to 1975. In contrast, the CSPI story cited only studies conducted prior to 1972.

I would like to put the argument this way: At the very least, there is strong evidence *on the scientific level* that the matter is in doubt. Let's leave out the "conspiratorial" level. Now, shouldn't the general, theoretical arguments decide the issue? Let me list some:

1. Other countries and other societies have high-cholesterol diets yet little heart disease (North India, Japan, France; Eskimos, Yemenites) *relative to the United States.*

2. Other countries and other societies have low-cholesterol diets yet have heart disease relatively higher than in the United States (World War II prisoners of war, the island of St. Helena, Trappist monks, the Gujrati of Kenya). These and the above examples may sound like obscure cases, but there are numerous supporting population studies.

3. Heart disease remains the number-one cause of death in the United States, despite the promotion of low-cholesterol diets for some twenty-five years.

4. Nineteenth-century Americans had a butter- and milk-rich diet and little atherosclerosis. Were they dying from other causes *before* heart disease claimed them? Not likely: death from heart disease today quite often comes at an age younger than that common to death from our ancestors' diseases.

5. In all of history, there is no comparable indictment of natural foods such as eggs and milk. A general appreciation of nature and our evolution would indicate the folly of such ready-made scapegoats. As Linus Pauling says, "We must educate people away from the dangerous idea that you can control heart disease by not eating foods such as eggs, butter, and milk. This oversimplified idea is totally wrong."

6. The foods that tend to replace eggs and dairy products have dangers of their own that are becoming increasingly evident. To my mind it is enough to note that *trans*-fats and poly-

unsaturates have now been found out as villains in their own right. Yet at any large American hospital one is likely to be served a cream substitute containing hydrogenated oil and simulated egg yolks!

I would like to offer these six broad considerations to anyone who hasn't the time or the opportunity to study the controlled scientific experiments. Perhaps this is more convincing than the Bassler first rule ("You can eat anything that's alive!").

THE PARSLEY PRINCIPLE

Well, such critics of the egg as CSPI say, "Peas surpass eggs as a source of iron, thiamin, niacin, and vitamin C. . . . Calorie for calorie, green peas supply similar amounts of total protein, calcium, phosphorus, Vitamin A, and riboflavin." Their cry is, Let them eat peas!

It's understandable that nutritionists are continually looking for substitutes for this and that. The danger is, the numbers game is very deceptive simply because (1) nutrients work together, synergistically, and (2) we don't really know a fraction of the values in foods. Sure, peas have more vitamin C. (Eggs have virtually none!) Parsley also is an excellent source of the vitamin—and no book on nutrition fails to mention this fact. But just how practical is it to try to get good nutrition by reading food values?

"Calorie for calorie" means that you'd have to eat about seven or eight ounces of green peas to equal one medium egg. That's most of a package of frozen peas, hardly a reasonable serving. It's also about thirty cents' worth, against eight cents for the egg. Again, a matter of practicalities. Unfortunately, butter is two or three times the cost of margarine—an exception to the general rule that whole foods are also cheaper foods.

It's nice to sprinkle parsley on your salads and vegetables. It's also a natural way of combating bad breath. But parsley is a poor way, practically speaking, to get the vitamin C you need.

THE WHOLE LIFE DIET STANDS
FOR WHOLE FOODS AND THE
WHOLE EGG!

It's true that the American Heart Association hasn't asked us to cut eggs out completely: three a week is their recommendation. It's also true that they've recently added aerobic exercise to their prescription for a healthy heart. What I object to is the extremism in nutrition that the egg recommendation leads to.

All of a sudden we have egg-yolk substitutes, of dubious pedigree. On CSPI's "Nutrition Scoreboard," eggs and milk products receive negative values! A recipe book put out by the AHA fails to list eggs at all! Imitation ice creams, containing hydrogenated oils, are recommended instead of ice cream made with honest-to-goodness milk.

I don't ask you to believe Tom Bassler. Examine the evidence. If it's contradictory, think about the nature of food. Whole foods—all of them—are the key to life; whatever has the power to grow has the power to help you grow.

SEVEN

Megavitamins, Micronutrients, and the "Balanced Diet"

Second only to the cholesterol controversy in confusion is the megavitamin flap. Can we make a reasoned decision about taking vitamin and mineral supplements?

The term *mega* just means "great," "large," or "a million." When it is used in *megavitamin* it can mean many things to many people. I use the term when a vitamin becomes a conspicuous part of the diet. Some common symptoms are associated with a *distortion* of the nutrient balance: imbalances between needs for certain nutrients and their intake. Any time you distort your diet, you should review possible hazards and weigh them against possible benefit. Death is a clear possibility when it comes to distorting nutrient intake.

TAKING VITAMIN PILLS CAN BE DANGEROUS: START WITH THAT!

If you have pills around the house, read the labels and see if there is potential toxic effect from overdose. Almost any drug obtained by prescription can be dangerous; that's why they are available only by prescription. Many of the over-the-counter drugs are also dangerous when taken in large amounts. Aspirin, for example, is one of the leading causes of death-by-overdose in children. A large bottle of aspirin can kill almost anyone. That's why we have these new bottle caps that take a genius to open. When a child is old enough to open the cap, he should also be smart enough not to eat the entire contents.

Having worked in a medical examiner's office, I am aware of the hazards of many common household items. Even bleach and detergents have taken their toll. One of the most dangerous things I can think of is the use of empty pop bottles to store leftover liquids that are poisonous. It is only a matter of time before a small child will wander in, pick up the bottle, and sample the contents.

What has this to do with vitamins?

Many vitamins come in attractive colors and flavors. They are available in bulk. Millions of households store shelves of these pills, and there are magazine articles encouraging their use every day. Children see adults taking the pretty pills; so it is not surprising to hear of an overdose occasionally.

How much of a hazard are vitamin pills, really? That varies with the contents of the pill. I consider pills with iron, vitamin A, and vitamin D to be potentially dangerous, and I store them with the same care as other hazardous items. I advise people to avoid pills containing these nutrients, unless there is a clear need for them. (I do not think we need a multivitamin with iron, A, or D for routine use.)

Let's consider the characteristics of these three.

Vitamin A

Stimson of Seattle wrote a review of vitamin A intoxication in adults, and Shaywitz and associates reported a case in a child.[1] The FDA used to limit the amount of vitamin A to 10,000 IU per pill; but these individuals were taking much more than that. One man had symptoms in a month on 1,000,000 IU per day, while 50,000 IU caused symptoms in three years in another man. All suffered from fatigue, some needing daily naps. All had pain in bones and joints; sometimes the pain was very severe. Some showed loss of hair, occasionally loss of eyebrows. Treatment included abruptly stopping the intake of vitamin A, and all improved quickly. Naps were no longer needed after a few days off the vitamin, and by two weeks all of the patients felt relatively normal.*

Toxicity takes time at these doses, because the vitamin has to be stored in body fat until dangerous levels are reached. However, acute poisoning can follow a serving of polar-bear liver with 4,000,000 IU. But who do you know who might eat polar-bear liver? No one. Those who live in the Arctic know that it is poisonous, so they wouldn't be serving it anyway. However, the comparison is valid if we look into the vitamin bottle. How many pills equal a serving of polar-bear liver? If the pills contain the FDA's limit of 10,000 IU, we have to worry about someone swallowing 400 pills, not very likely unless they were candy-coated and served up during a double-feature movie. Even then, it would be a heroic amount of pill-taking! If "mega-vitamin A" pills contained twenty times the RDA, then only 40 pills would equal a serving of polar-bear liver—and 40 pills is not an unusual intake for a child if the pills are pretty and candy coated. Therefore, I suggest we all read labels, and avoid pills with vitamin A unless they are prescribed.

Natural sources of vitamin A include the yellow and bright green vegetables. Their color is due to *carotenes*, substances our own bodies convert to vitamin A. Artificial sources include fortified milk. The yellow color of cow's cream is due to carotenes. Goat's milk is white because the carotenes are converted to colorless vitamin A. The yellow color of egg yolk and cheese also reflects carotenes from the diet of the chicken and the cow. Our bodies store vitamin A and carotenes in our fat for very long times, and it is almost impossible to find anyone deficient in this vitamin unless they have had a medical problem that gives them trouble in digesting and absorbing fat.

---

* Under the careful supervision of doctors, vitamin A in *emulsion* form has been used with success and safety in treating specific conditions. Here we're concerned only with uninformed, general use in pill form, as part of a preventive program.

You will notice that this fat-soluble vitamin is present in *both* animal and vegetable sources. In animal sources (egg yolk, cream, etc.) it is associated with cholesterol, so when you go on a "low cholesterol" diet you reduce your natural intake of this and other "fat-soluble" vitamins. Vegetable sources for vitamin A are more than adequate *if* they are eaten. In fact, some vegetarians actually have a yellow tinge to their skin and serum because of the heavy load of carotenes from their diet of plant materials.

By the way, carrots aren't necessarily a good source of carotene and vitamin A. In raw form, the carotene is within indigestible cell walls. Cooked carrots provide some 5 to 20 percent of the carotene for nutrition—a rare case of cooked being better than raw.

Vitamin D

The FDA suggests that we need only 400 IU of vitamin D; and I agree. I worry about artificial sources in the diet, such as fortified milk (which contains about 400 IU per quart) because there are some animal studies showing that added vitamin D can cause atherosclerosis. Oddly enough, skim milk has the natural vitamin D removed with the cream (supposedly to reduce cholesterol intake and protect against atherosclerosis) and then artificial vitamin D is added—making me worry about the *D* causing atherosclerosis!

So, I prefer whole raw milk without the added vitamin D.

We can make our own vitamin D by exposing our skin to the ultraviolet rays in sunshine. Human pigment levels adjust to keep the daily synthesis within physiological limits. White skin allows deep penetration of ultraviolet light and maximal synthesis of the vitamin. Racial pigmentation may be a genetic adaptation to the available sunlight. Dark skin blocks some of the tropical sunlight and keeps vitamin D production within limits. Even white skin gets dark in the summer—a tan that limits vitamin D formation.

Foods rich in vitamin D include the "oily fish" (sardines, salmon, and herring), egg yolk, liver, mushrooms, and green plants.

Vitamin D is vital for calcium balance and bone metabolism. Extra intake from supplements should be given to children who are growing fast—especially during the winter months—at a dose of 400 IU. The elderly who can't get out into the sun need the vitamin also. Average healthy Americans who exercise in sunlight can use their tanning skin as an indication that they do not need extra vitamin D. However, smog and ordinary window glass may block out the ultraviolet rays, increasing your need for the vitamin.

Toxic symptoms can appear when massive doses are given (in the range of 10,000 IU per pound of body weight). A hundred-pound human given 1,000,000 IU per day could have headaches, vomiting, fractures, kidney stones, elevated cholesterol levels and high blood pressure, with calcium deposits in kidneys and other tissues of the body. If pills are limited to 400 IU each, they are safe. No one can eat 2,500 pills per day!

Iron

There is good evidence that 1,000 mg of elemental iron can cause death in toddlers. Any package that contains 500 mg iron should be treated as a potential poison, with the proper precautions of storage. The pills with 60 mg iron, *ferrous sulphate,* are clearly iron pills, but there are many other vitamin tablets that also contain iron. These may contain 250 tablets per bottle; and the tablets may be colored and flavored to resemble candy! This explains why iron-containing compounds ranked third in the United States among drugs responsible for fatal poisonings in children under the age of five years, in 1973.

The smallest dose to cause death is about 200 mg iron, but there have been recoveries with overdoses as high as 15 grams (15,000 mg). Such massive doses are highly corrosive, destroying the lining of the stomach, so that reparative surgery is often required if the toddler survives. Symptoms are dramatic: bloody diarrhea and vomiting. This can be followed by collapse, coma, and death in less than twenty-four hours.

Since fatalities are possible from as few as four iron pills, adults should make every effort to keep them away from children. The best way is to keep them out of the house completely!

When supplemental iron is needed, it should be treated like any other dangerous household item and used only when indicated; the excess should be discarded promptly.

But who *does* need iron? Crosby estimates that 10 percent of menstruating women need extra iron.[2] Elderly people who have lost their teeth may not be able to eat iron-rich foods. In one report from Missouri, 10 percent of the women and 20 percent of the men over age fifty-nine were iron-deficient.[3] However, replacement iron should be on an individual basis. Mandatory iron "fortification" of too many foods may cause dangerous iron overload in some individuals. This can cause serious damage to the liver and other organs.

LOOK FIRST TO WHOLE FOODS, AND ONLY THEN TO PILLS

Obviously, vitamins A and D as well as iron are dangerous in pill form. So, every effort should be made to obtain these vital nutrients from whole, natural sources.

For example, the daily requirement of 400 IU for vitamin D is contained in one ounce of herring or mackerel, two ounces of canned sardines, or three ounces of tuna or salmon. Other sources include egg yolk, butter, and liver. Using food instead of pills is more natural—and safer. Small children cannot overdose on herring!

Iron is so plentiful in a normal mixed diet that a man is rarely anemic unless he is bleeding. The cause of his bleeding is far more important than his iron deficiency. The same is true of women who are not menstruating. It would be wrong to give these individuals iron without tracking down the cause of the bleeding.

Self-medication with iron for symptoms of fatigue and dizziness is probably a useless effort. Elwood found that these symptoms were not related to iron levels.[4] He examined thousands of women in Wales, treated those with low iron, and found that the symptoms did not change as the blood counts returned to normal. He learned that anemia did not cause symptoms until hemoglobin levels were below 8 gm/dl (the normal level is over 12 gm/dl for women).

It would be silly to discuss the megavitamin use of the fat-soluble vitamins A and D. They are so dangerous in pill form and so plentiful in our American diet that overdose is far more common than deficiency problems. In the rare case where large doses of these nutrients are needed, physicians can prescribe them. Rickets, a bone disease caused by lack of vitamin D, can be *prevented* by only 400 IU per day; but once it appears, it is *treated* with 10,000 IU per day for a month or two. However, giving 10,000 IU to a normal child is very hazardous. The casual over-the-counter pill should not contain such massive doses.

ARE MEGAVITAMINS THE ANSWER
TO EMPTY CALORIES?

If processed food lacks something, it seems logical to put it back. A slice of off-the-shelf white bread has shortening. It can be toasted and spread with margarine. Shortening and margarine contain dangerous *trans*-fat, known to cause atherosclerosis in animals. Is there anything that can "protect" against this piece of toast?

No! *Trans*-fat is capable of causing heart disease without any associated deficiency. I'm repeating myself—but it bears repeating.

You bake up a huge sugary cake at home—no shortening, but a lot of white pastry flour and white sugar. Is there anything that can protect you from 300 calories of homemade cake?

Yes. The cake has "empty calories" but no toxic substances. You can replace what was removed from the flour and sugar in refining them: wheat germ, wheat-germ oil, vitamin E, cereal bran, amino acids, and water-soluble vitamins.

Enter now the health nut who thinks in terms of chemicals and pills. He knows that empty calories lurk everywhere, so he starts his day with a handful of pills and capsules. Pectin and bran come in tablets now. Brewer's yeast contains B vitamins and amino acids. Wheat-germ oil and vitamin C come in capsules. The one-a-day vitamin has a little of everything.

DUMB!

The pill-taking health nut has made the most common mistake I have seen—trusting an industry for nourishment. The food industry *first* makes a palatable product that sells at a profit, *then* gives some thought to the health benefits, adding whatever nutrients look good on the package. The vitamin industry does the same thing. It packages whatever the public is buying. Whenever a government agency comes out with new guidelines for nutrition, a pill quickly appears on the shelf with a similar content. The pill is there to meet the demand. The pill is not alive, and there is no connection between your needs and the pill's contents except the profit the industry hopes to make. The same can be said for processed food: a package's first duty is to *profit,* not nutrition! Don't trust anyone. Eat only living things! These are strong words, but the illusion that added vitamins have solved our modern empty-calorie problems is impossible to dispel without straight talk.

Now let's go back and look at that cake with the empty calories again. Read the recipe. You don't have to worry about any whole foods in the recipe, like whole milk, eggs, whole-wheat flour, or fruit. If you grind your own flour you will have all the bran, wheat germ, and wheat-germ oil needed to cover the flour calories.

But a cake has some white flour and sugar; add up those empty calories. Look at the frosting too—more white sugar. Even a homemade cake will contain 33 percent empty calories. If you eat it, you will "owe yourself" the missing EFAs, silicon, and vitamin C.

At the end of each day, think back over the empty calories you ate—snacks at work, a pastry here, a sugary drink there, all the treats that covered a missing meal. Is there anything that can be done to correct the problem at night?

First, the empty calories can't be removed without exercise; and you can't exercise without nutrients—so the dilemma compounds itself. You must exercise to burn off excess calories, and at the same time take more calories in the nourishing whole foods to match the deficiency.

Let's say the day was a nutritional mess: 600 calories of empty food. You missed breakfast, and substituted a prune Danish plus coffee with cream and sugar. A snack for lunch; white toast with bacon, lettuce, and tomato, plus coffee again. Now it is supper. You are home and your nutrition is under your control. Nothing can be done about the grease in the bacon or the *trans*-fat in the ordinary white bread. However, the bread, pastry, and sugar have given you about 600 empty calories. This can be fixed:

Exercise to burn off the bad 600 calories: jog an hour or walk two hours—six miles.

Fiber from half a cup of bran will give silicon. (Just add boiling water to half a cup of cereal bran, wait five minutes, and eat with a spoon. Or add soft bran to a supper dish: soup, vegetables, or cereal.)

EFAs from nuts, seeds, or whole grain. Sunflower seeds can be bought in bulk and stored in the refrigerator.

Vitamin B complex, in yeast, yogurt, or wheat germ. Store wheat germ in the refrigerator. I like to use yogurt plus sunflower seeds as a routine source of both EFAs and the B complex.

Vitamin C, one gram, plus a piece of raw fruit.

Protein, the daily intake of one serving of egg, chicken, fish, or lean meat will meet protein requirements.

Now let's take a closer look at the vitamins that seem to be so useful.

VITAMIN C—EVERYBODY'S FAVORITE

Is Extra Vitamin C Needed?

Let's look at the aerobic athlete who decides *not* to take extra vitamin C. If he lives in a warm climate where fresh fruit is available all the time, he can cover each mile he jogs with a whole orange or the equivalent. Six miles, six oranges. Two pounds of raw fruit and vegetables contain about a gram of vitamin C—enough for a normal day. Man was designed to live like this, and many Tarahumara Indians can run marathon distances in the mountains of Mexico without any extra vitamin C in the form of the ascorbic-acid tablets so common in the American gym bags.

What happens to the athlete when it snows? There is no *real* fresh fruit in the supermarket in the winter. Shipping takes time. After the fruit is picked, it starts to lose vitamins. When orange juice is pasteurized it loses 50 percent of its biologically available vitamin C. Old produce has even less vitamin C. How can the athlete adjust? First, he can reduce his exercise. Winter can be a time to rest, to turn to less stressful activities.

What if the athlete continues to train hard when his diet contains less ascorbic acid? Cravings for fresh produce are a clue to falling blood levels of vitamin C. Aches and pains mean tissue levels are low. Flu symptoms are a warning that he can no longer handle stress. Winter colds are due to a drop in dietary ascorbic acid plus the stress of colder weather. Once the cold appears, the severity of the symptoms depends on how deficient the diet is; less ascorbic acid means more discomfort.[5]

Most of us carry around enough tissue vitamin C for about seventy hard workouts—for joggers, any run that exceeds a third of the weekly mileage is probably stressful. When these hard workouts add up to seventy, you will have used up your stored vitamin C and will feel pain.

So when are megadoses of vitamin C called for?

When Dr. Mollen polled physicians with over ten marathons under their belts he found that 95 percent agreed that megadoses of viamin C were important in marathon training. (Only 50 percent of physicians who ran fewer than ten marathons thought it was important!)

How much is a megadose?

Dr. Man-Li S. Yew studied the effects of vitamin C on young animals: growth rate, healing rate, and ability to handle the stress of surgery.[6] The best results were seen at doses that translated to a human dose of ten grams per day. Human studies on twins also suggest the same benefits, with doses of only a gram a day. One group showed an increased growth of about half an inch with vitamin C. Both twins were healthy, but the one on ascorbic acid grew faster. Patients with bed sores were also tested. The sores healed twice as fast in patients given ascorbic acid.[7]

The Runner's Eighteen-Month Test for Vitamin C

If you don't take a gram of ascorbic acid each day, when will you get injured?

If you can get fresh fruit and vegetables every day, no injury can be predicted, because your diet will keep your tissue levels high. However, if part of your diet is processed and part of your produce is "old" (i.e., shipped great distances), then start adding up the hard workouts. Seventy hard workouts usually take about eighteen months. Many beginners train and race well for eighteen months; then the pains start. They try stretching, yoga, orthotics, and injections; but nothing can be expected to work if tissue ascorbic acid levels are low. Under the microscope, the early injuries look like regional scurvy—tissue fibers turn to mush and fall apart. Good tissue, collagen, has the strength of steel, fiber for fiber, and it can become stronger with training by laying down more fibers. However, poor tissue just falls apart by itself. Poor tissue is usually low in silicon, vitamin C, or protein. If you don't take vitamin C, you should rest about three months each year, to allow your diet to build up your body stores of vitamin C. If you want to race every month of every year, you must keep your dietary vitamin C very high—about a gram for each ten kilometers.

Vitamin C and Cancer

I think we will find that high tissue levels of vitamin C will prevent many diseases. Human studies cannot be done for some of these conditions, for many reasons, but animal studies already suggest that vitamin C prevents cancer.

Carcinogens cause cancer by damaging chromosomes. When human white blood cells were incubated with a carcinogen, chromosomal breakage was observed in a test tube. Adding vitamin C reduced the number of breaks by 31.7 percent.[8] I interpret this to mean that high tissue levels of vitamin C reduce our chances of getting cancer! This study was done at the Cleveland Clinic in the Department of Hematology by Dr. Shamberger and others, and presented by Dr. Linus Pauling, March 7, 1973.

Pauling has also been involved in other studies suggesting that vitamin C protects us from cancer.[9] It has been suggested for prevention of bladder tumors.[10]

Weisburger encourages eating salads with main meals as a way of keeping the vitamin C intake high enough to block the hazards of nitrosamines.[11] Salads give our diet a high vitamin C content when fresh produce is in season; however, carcinogens like nitrosamines are present the year round. Seasonal exposure to carcinogens should be matched with high vitamin C intake; therefore I take at least a gram of vitamin C every day.

Ewan Cameron, a Scottish surgeon, suggests that large doses of vitamin C would help patients with advanced cancer. He reported a series of fifty patients who were treated with large doses of ascorbic acid. They were suffering with advanced cancer at the time the ascorbic acid was started. All were already being treated with the conventional surgery and other medications, so the extra vitamin C was just added to their therapy. Cameron's theory focuses on the material around the cancer cell called "ground substance." If the ground substance is tough, the cancer cell has a hard time growing. He theorizes that vitamin C slows down the tumor growth by keeping the ground substance intact.[12]

Cameron and Pauling found that vitamin C (usually 10 gm/day) increased survival times for "hopeless" cancer patients in Scotland.[13] About 90 percent of the patients on vitamin C lived three times longer than controls who had similar tumors, but did not get megavitamin C. Interestingly, about 10 percent of the patients on vitamin C lived much longer—over twenty times longer than the controls! Because megavitamin C is so free from side effects, I'd like to see similar studies done outside of Scotland to see if the same benefit results.

Vitamin C and the Cardiovascular System

When I review the autopsy slides on an athlete who has died of atherosclerosis, I look first at the inner lining of the arteries for the pavement-lining cells—called *endothelial* cells. These fall off when vitamin C levels are low.[14] I expect them to be absent in cases of progressive atherosclerosis. As you will recall from Chapter Five, this is one of the mechanisms by which the artery fills up with blood clots; when the endothelial cells come off, clots are attracted to the area. Athletes with low levels of vitamin C usually also have weak Achilles tendons or joint cartilage, limiting athletic performance. For this reason I do not expect to find marathon runners with progressive atherosclerosis, since the same weakness that damaged their arteries would also damage their bones and joints.

In an article in *Lancet*, Taylor reviews the relationship between low levels of vitamin C and stroke.[15] He paints a grim picture for those who are getting inadequate supplies of the vitamin. Their blood vessels weaken and degenerate as their blood levels of vitamin C fall. Diabetics seem to suffer most; they appear to need more vitamin C to keep their vessels healthy.

Spittle has been saying for years that vitamin C raises cholesterol levels.[16] She thought the elevation was from the bad cholesterol leaving the arteries, making them healthier. This was before the discovery of friendly HDL-cholesterol! Now we know that Spittle was right. Patients with atherosclerosis do improve with increased tissue levels of the vitamin. The rising HDL-cholesterol is associated with protection against heart attack.[17] Spittle knew this ten years ago; there were fewer deaths among patients who took vitamin C.

Vitamin C and the Bladder

Gout can be helped with vitamin C also. When the patient with gout eats too many animal products, he produces too much uric acid. To understand how this works, we should remember the metabolism of birds. Birds must be lightweight to fly, so they do not have bladders full of urine. They put up waste nitrogen products in a paste, a white chalky material full of *uric acid*. Earthbound mammals, on the other hand, can afford the luxury of bladders. So they transform their nitrogen waste into *urea*, a very soluble molecule found in urine. Unfortunately, some humans have trouble with this metabolic pathway and they make too much uric acid—the substance birds produce. When humans have too much uric acid, it crystallizes out in bones, joints, and kidneys, causing much pain; that is, they have gout.

If you have gout and start taking vitamin C, it will cause an increased excretion of uric acid.[18] In the long run, this is good, because it will lower your tissue levels of uric acid and probably prevent the pain of gout attacks. However, when you start taking the vitamin there will be a sudden increase of uric acid in the urine—increasing the risk of uric-acid stones in the kidney. I try to match my intake of vitamin C with enough fluids to keep my urine clear. For runners, the risk of stones goes up because of the dehydration associated with sweat loss. My rule is: *Drink whatever you have to so you produce a quart of clear urine each day.* This usually means a pint of beer for each ten kilometers (six miles).

Vitamin C also increases another material in the urine that can cause stones in some people. Oxalates are the most common form of kidney stones. All vegetable foods contain oxalates, and there is a steady excretion of oxalates in your urine all the time. However, some people handle vitamin C badly, and it causes higher levels of urine oxalates. Running dehydration adds to the risk of high-urine oxalates; so again—one pint of beer for each ten kilometers.

Vitamin C doesn't *cause* kidney stones, but it *helps* some people form them.

Last, But Not Least—Vitamin C and the Common Cold!

The popularity of megadoses of vitamin C began in 1970, when Linus Pauling published his book *Vitamin C and the Common Cold.* I have been using a gram of ascorbic acid each day since. If I feel a cold coming on I follow Pauling's advice and take a gram an hour, up to ten grams a day.

This same idea was used by Dr. Terry Anderson of Toronto. He found a 30 percent "protection" against days of disability due to the virus. Dr. Anderson's study involved 407 subjects using the vitamin and 411 using a placebo (a pill with no vitamin activity, but the same flavor and color). Therefore, I think the vitamin does have a real nutritional effect against cold symptoms. I suspect it helps our bodies fight off the virus. Many of us carry around a number of viruses all the time, but the virus doesn't do anything to us when our resistance is high. But as soon as we are exhausted or weakened . . . *wham!* Three days later, the home-bred virus is all over us—or a new virus can attack us.

Hazards of Aspirin with Vitamin C

Whenever aspirin is taken, a small blood loss occurs. The more aspirin you take, the more blood you lose from your gut. Even if the aspirin is given in your vein, there is a little blood loss in the gut. However, when you combine aspirin with vitamin C, then you can get a large hemorrhage. In a study done on rats, there was no blood loss with vitamin C alone.[19] Aspirin is also dangerous in anyone with a bleeding problem of any kind.

Let Your Stress Load Tell You When to
Take More than a Gram

Stress of any kind increases our need for ascorbic acid. Jet lag, missing a night's sleep, running a marathon, giving a talk to a strange audience, fighting with a loved one—any physical or emotional stress increases the need for the vitamin.

Smoking lowers blood levels of vitamin C.[20]

Contraceptive pills lower vitamin C.[21]

Surgery causes a drop too.[22]

Spittle has suggested that vitamin C prevents blood clots in veins; and women who smoke and take birth control pills were found to have a high risk of clots. I think that vitamin C may be the common denominator, since both the pill and smoking lower it.

Using the formula of one gram for every ten kilometers, you would need about ten grams to run a hundred kilometers. That seems about right; however, I usually take five grams a day for the three days after a hundred-kilometer run also. I feel I've been stressed by the run, and the stress lasts for three days.

Does Vitamin C Improve Racing Performance?

If you count getting to the starting line as part of performance, yes! Many of the runners who train without vitamin C will get the flu during the week before the big race. Flu symptoms are just an index of stress. Vitamin C helps protect against stress, and the virus. If you don't show up at the start of the race, you don't have any performance to talk about! Vitamin C helps you get there.

Does Vitamin C Prevent Injuries?

It helps you make tougher tissue during training, so you can handle bigger work loads. This takes six weeks. It helps prevent "overuse" injury by giving you a stronger body to use. It does not, of course, protect against accidents like stepping in a hole.

THE VITAMIN B COMPLEX

When Megavitamins Have Immediate, Observable Results: The B-Complex "Flush"

The *niacin flush* is a drug-induced, pink-faced feeling of well-being resulting from an expensive injection containing niacin (nicotinic acid). It is an effectve tool for certain types of headache. Also, since the flushing is caused by dilation of blood vessels, it can be used for a variety of conditions associated with narrowed vessels: spasm of arteries, varicose and decubitus ulcers, anginal chest pain, peripheral arteriosclerosis, etc.

I use the term *thiamin flush* for a washing out or saturation of the body tissues with the vitamin B complex from *food* sources. Among other things, it's a good answer for depression. There isn't enough thiamin in foods to produce the itching and burning sensation caused by nicotinic acid; however, the pink-faced feeling of well-being *can* be induced with exercise and foods.

When this euphoria is brought on with dietary manipulation, all that is required is a "loading dose" of a cup of yogurt and a tablespoon of wheat germ or fresh-ground whole-wheat flour each day for four or five days. Add cereal bran to each meal to give the yogurt organism a good supply of gut fiber in which to grow. This will saturate your tissues with the B-complex vitamins. They are water-soluble, and cannot be overdosed, as excess is lost through the kidneys. If your diet is otherwise well-balanced, any surplus of the B-complex group will produce a feeling of well-being, the so-called *thiamin flush*.

Brewer's yeast comes as tablets and powder. Read the label. Ten grams of yeast contains about 1.5 mg thiamin. That much is contained in fifteen of the ten-gram tablets. To adhere to the "whole food" concept of my philosophy on diet, *you have to reconstitute brewer's yeast by adding what has been removed in processing—the beer!* Drink a pint of cheap local draft beer (no preservatives) with ten grams of brewer's yeast.

Jog or walk at least three miles a day. This demand for energy stimulates the mitochondria to use thiamin and the other B-complex vitamins in the foods. The brain runs on carbohydrate energy, and the little mitochondria are the engines that burn carbohydrate. They are nothing more than protein envelopes of enzymes, and *enzymes* is another word for the vitamin B-complex group in the body.

This combination of thiamin-rich foods and a little exercise creates a metabolic "high" that works wonders for the usual type of depression. The thiamin flush can happen at any hour. You may awaken at five A.M., alert and enthusiastic, with warm fingers, toes, ears, and nose. You will feel like exercising and you will burn more calories that day. This is a good tool during any weight-loss effort.

When the jogging is increased to six miles a day, the benefits are large enough to measure in depressed patients under the care of a psychiatrist. Thaddeus Kostrubala has advocated this diet and running therapy in his book *The Joy of Running.* I have met some of his patients, and they're the best evidence for me that he's on the right track.

Pep Up a Friend with Brewer's Yeast and a Beer!

If you have a friend who would like to get up in the morning and jog with you, but he tells you he is "too tired" to get out of bed, give him the formula for a thiamin flush. But be sure to warn him not to run too hard. Several joggers I know have felt too enthusiastic, jumped out of bed, run too fast, and hurt something. No matter how good you feel, you still must build up your mileage slowly—adding no more than a mile a month to the maximum distance you run.

Remember, put the beer back with the yeast for a natural

thiamin flush! The whole foods are better than a vitamin pill. The yeast plus beer make a whole food—all the vitamins, amino acids, and trace elements that the yeast needed are present. You know that you are taking a living food source, and you don't have to trust the vitamin industry. Ten grams of yeast has about five grams of protein, too. However, it is too expensive to count it as a protein source, since you'd need about a hundred grams of brewer's yeast a day to meet protein requirements. (Remember the "parsley principle.")

VITAMIN B_{12}

Vitamin B_{12} is a vitamin with cobalt in it. It's found in animal products, both meat and dairy, and it's important for all the cells of the body. Inadequate levels of B_{12} cause anemia and brain damage. Pure vegetarians can get into trouble if they don't eat an occasional egg or piece of cheese. It is very important for vegetarian mothers to get extra vitamin B_{12} while they are pregnant and when they are nursing. If I were a vegetarian, I'd use eggs and dairy products for the needed B_{12}; they are more natural than pills. However, it's important to realize that infants have a critical need for adequate B_{12} and that it cannot be met using milk from a pure-vegetarian mother. Infants raised without this vitamin can die.[23] If the mother does want to avoid animal products, she can obtain synthetic vitamin B_{12} (cyanocobalamin).[24]

Many people still think that megavitamin C destroys vitamin B_{12}. It doesn't, but it interferes with the *test* for B_{12} in the test tube. Victor Herbert (the genius in the lab, not the composer) pointed out that blood from individuals taking large doses of vitamin C cannot be tested for vitamin B_{12} unless a special step is taken during the procedure. Before this was known, it appeared the ascorbic acid could destroy vitamin B_{12}, because whenever the two were present together, the levels of B_{12} appeared to be low. Just an artifact in the lab; nothing to worry about! However, if you are taking megadoses of ascorbic acid and you do happen to have your vitamin B_{12} level measured, and it is low, be sure your doctor knows about Herbert's report so he can check the lab method used.[25]

VITAMIN E—SEX VITAMIN, LONGEVITY VITAMIN, PLACEBO?

Track coaches were giving vitamin E to sprinters decades ago. Like anything else with vague benefits, it was claimed to help you live and love longer! Consider:

Buck was in his fifties. He had recovered from his first heart attack well enough. He had stopped smoking and tried to improve his diet and exercise habits, but he continued having chest pain. A friend told him to try vitamin E. This was a popular over-the-counter treatment in Canada during the late 1960s. Buck took 1,000 IU of vitamin E each day. His chest pain lessened "almost at once," and he began walking great distances. Now, over ten years later, he is a marathon runner. He still takes megavitamin E, and swears that his chest pain comes back whenever he stops the vitamin.

There are a lot of cases like Buck's. But whenever a controlled study is done, using placebo (empty) pills, scientists fail to show that vitamin E helps—at least not so you'd notice statistically.

My job was to talk with Buck and formulate a story for a magazine piece—did the vitamin help? Could it help? Why?

Buck is one of those heavy-bearded fellows with muscular shoulders. He likes pretty girls. While we were talking, a pretty girl jogged by. He had to stop and watch—commenting on her hair, her legs, her smile. After she had passed, he picked up our conversation again. Yes, it was true, he swore by megadoses of vitamin E. Just recently, on a trip to an out-of-town marathon, he had forgotten his vitamin. The pain returned, and he had to find a drugstore in a strange town—and buy enough E to get him back home.

At first, I thought Buck was using vitamin E as a crutch—sort of a placebo. If it wasn't there, his anxiety would produce the pain. That sounded logical. But I was wrong. As soon as I went to his home, my eyes were opened—in two ways!

I knew I had a logical explanation for Buck's dependence on vitamin E when I met his wife. She was a chain-smoker! She quickly filled the air around us with tobacco smoke—so that I would have been absorbing the equivalent of one cigarette per hour if I had stayed there. The smoke burned my eyes immediately, and began to irritate the lining of my nose. It was obvious that Buck's use of vitamin E was just a defense against smoke. With all those oxides in the air, he needed a high-tissue level of antioxidants to protect himself; and vitamin E is a good antioxidant! This is especially important for heart patients, because it protects the small blood vessels and platelets so that the secondhand smoke doesn't cause clots.

If vitamin E worked for Buck, why did it fail to show a benefit when it was used in a large controlled study of cardiac patients?

Buck was using an antioxidant (E) for protection against a specific oxidizing agent (tobacco smoke). I am sure that it would show some benefits under those conditions, but how many cardiac patients would want to live with a chain-smoker to find out?

Will vitamin E help a patient who does not live with a smoker?

Perhaps. There are a number of theories, and I am open-minded on the subject. Vitamin E seems safe enough. I would use it just for the placebo effect; anxiety is real, and anything you can do to lessen it will help.

Farrell and Bieri reported no toxic side effects when 28 adults took between 100 IU and 800 IU per day for three years.[26] About half of the volunteers reported vague benefits. A number of screening lab tests were done, and no abnormalities could be found. This suggests that most people can take up to 800 IU safely.

Smog and Blood Clots: Studies Show Vitamin E Protects against Oxide

Animals receiving twice the RDA of vitamin E were protected against ozone (the oxidant in photochemical smog). They were compared to animals getting the same amount of vitamin E that the average American gets—less than half of the RDA. The animal study was reported by Mustafa, with the obvious piece of advice that humans living in smog would be smart if they tried to get a high level of vitamin E in their diet.[27] This is the mechanism by which Buck's megavitamin E protected him from his wife's secondhand smoke.

Animals fed antioxidants (vitamins C and E, and BHT, about which you'll read more later) were protected against skin cancer.[28] The cancer was induced in 24 percent of the hairless mice who were not getting the antioxidants; none of the mice on antioxidants developed tumors. Skin cancer is caused by ultraviolet light, which penetrates the tissue where it photo-oxidizes cholesterol into carcinogenic compounds. Hairless mice were exposed to the ultraviolet light for twenty-four weeks. Those receiving antioxidants were protected against the photo-oxidation!

Humans were fed 100 mg of d-a-tocopherol acetate (a form of vitamin E) each day for one week. Their red blood cells were protected against the effects of ozone intoxication in a test tube.[29] This suggests to me that the antioxidants play the same protective role in humans as in animals.

Steiner and Anastasi studied human platelets and suggested that vitamin E might be useful in preventing undesirable blood clots.[30] Rats deficient in vitamin E do get into trouble with sticky platelets, which could produce clots.[31]

Yes, Vitamin E Has Something to Do with Sex:
Men Need More of It!

Buck benefited from extra-large doses of vitamin E be-cause his diet was deficient. Most diets are very close to being deficient.[32] I object to having the RDA the same for males and females. It is well known that the need for vitamin E varies with the intake of unsaturated EFAs, and the need for EFAs in lower animals is about five to ten times higher for males than for females. Human males show five times the level of a urine metabolite of EFA that females do, suggesting that human males need five times the dietary intake of EFA.

Since vitamin E requirements are related to EFA intake, it is obvious that human men should need more than women. In fact, if Buck and his wife eat the same diet, the intake of vitamin E could be adequate for her and inadequate for him. They live together; the man gets the heart attack.

Karvonen of Helsinki worked with Turpeinen and others to show that added EFAs protected men from heart attack. One of the things they measured was the stickiness of the platelets (a factor in blood clots discussed in an earlier chapter). Men who were getting extra EFAs had healthier platelets.[33] This is understandable, since the membranes of platelets are rich in *phospholipids* with a high content of polyunsaturated fatty acids —the EFAs. This is a logical place for vitamin E to act if it is going to protect us from clots.

When I look at the heart muscle at autopsy, I try to find small areas where a clot has killed a muscle cell. People who die from coronary heart disease always have these, even if they don't die from a *myocardial infarction* (heart attack with dead muscle tissue). These small dead areas can cause sudden death by arrhythmia, or irregular heartbeat. Sticky platelets caused by low levels of EFAs or vitamin E deficiency could explain these small clots; so taking extra vitamin E could prevent this form of sudden death. It *is* logical!

How Much Vitamin E Is Enough?

The RDA used to be 30 IU and now is 15 IU per day. I think *human males need ten times more than the female*—from 150 to 300 IU per day. However, since vitamin E does occur naturally with the EFAs in seeds, nuts, and whole grains, there may be no need to take extra vitamin E by itself. On the other hand, if your intake of polyunsaturates is high, you do need more vitamin E to protect your tissues from oxides. Polyunsaturates that are extracted from seeds, nuts, and grains are probably deficient in vitamin E after the oil has been exposed to air, light, and time. Therefore, oils should be a bit suspect. Confusing, isn't it? The chant of the margarine promoters is "high in polyunsaturates."

What about Vitamin E for Atherosclerosis?

If the vitamin improves your fat—protecting EFAs, and making your body fat "friendlier"—then it could play a role in regression of atherosclerosis. However, that would take time—a long time, over a year. In one study using human males with narrowed vessels in their legs, vitamin E did not increase the blood flow to the legs until they had been taking it for twelve to eighteen months. After two years on the vitamin, the patients averaged a 34 percent increase in blood flow through the diseased arteries to the legs.[34] The dose was 300 milligrams of d-a-tocopherol acetate per day. Nevertheless, anyone with heart disease should look at both short- and long-term measures.

What about Vitamin E for Cancer?

Animal studies already prove the value of antioxidants in preventing cancer.[35] (Refer back to the vitamin C studies earlier in this chapter.) Humans who take it for this reason are logical. I doubt if anyone will use humans for such a study; it would take thirty years! In theory, any antioxidant would reduce your chances of getting cancer—vitamin C, vitamin E, and BHT. (BHT is a food additive. As we will see, just as polyunsaturates aren't necessarily good, so preservatives aren't necessarily bad.)

ESSENTIAL MINERALS AND
TRACE ELEMENTS

Things You Can Do with Megadoses of Silicon

Food fiber is rich in silicon. Alfalfa has ten times as much silicon as cereal bran. Bran has more silicon than pectin. And yet pectin is so good for you that "an apple a day keeps the doctor away!" * There is no RDA for silicon yet; however, we have done hair studies for silicon, discussed already in Chapter Three. The normal hair silicon levels are over 20 parts per million (ppm). Low levels, under 4 ppm, are associated with arthritis and atherosclerosis. You may have heard that alfalfa tea is good

---

* As we will see, folklore like this has been corroborated by scientific experiments and currently unfolding nutritional information.

for arthritis. Alfalfa has 12,000 ppm! The hard water that protected against heart attack (Chapter Three) has only about 10 ppm. Beer, with 35 ppm, also protects against heart attacks. To get megadoses of silicon, you just add alfalfa leaves to soups, salads, and tea.

How Does Silicon Work?

The silicon atom (Si) is used along with oxygen (O) to form a cross link with the hydrocarbon chain. The –O–Si–O– bonds add stability. Silicon is used in biology whenever strength is needed. Cereal bran is the armor that protects the seeds, remember. We use it in our skin, hair, and nails—our armor. It is found in chicken skin and cartilage (gristle), things that are not usually used for food. Gelatin, made from animal hooves, is rich in silicon—and can be used to make strong fingernails. (The hoof silicon becomes the nail silicon: armor!) Because "hard" things contain silicon, they have been systematically removed from our refined diet. That is unfortunate!

The importance of silicon is such a recent discovery that you won't find it even mentioned in the best nutrition books until the last few years. I predict that *silicon* will be the new "fad word" of the next decade—but it's so basic and so important that I welcome the fad!

When Should You Take Megadoses of Silicon?

Try it for symptoms of arthritis. If your knee or Achilles tendon feels about to break down, eat alfalfa for about six weeks. It takes six weeks to saturate the body with silicon and grow new tissue in the injured area. Minor twinges respond to both silicon and vitamin C. Both are needed for repair.

Can You Overdose on Alfalfa?

No. As we saw in Chapter Three, monkeys with atherosclerosis were given alfalfa as 50 percent of their diet, and the arteries cleared—even though 40 percent of their diet was fat, comparable to the average American diet! If monkeys can take a diet that is half alfalfa, I think humans can handle more than a little in their food.

Are There Other Sources of Silicon?

Maybe, but folklore has given us alfalfa. It has been in our dairy-food chain for thousands of years. I wouldn't trust a new source unless it had a similar history. Other sources include rice straw (rice straw tea has a long history of use also), hulls of all grains, and fruit pectins.

WHAT ABOUT OTHER MINERALS?

The more I read about minerals—the metals, salts, and other trace elements and micronutrients that are essential—the more convinced I am that we are designed by nature to eat living things. Alfalfa and cereal bran contain nice loads of the trace elements. If they are added to the diet regularly, you are keeping close to the soil. If pumpernickel or rye bread tastes unusually good, you may be getting the trace elements in molasses. Check the recipes for anything that tastes unusually good. Your taste buds may be telling you something.

Did you ever notice that a slice of buttered bread will always land sticky side down if you drop it? When that happened to me in front of an audience, I just picked it up, muttered something about "micronutrients," and continued making my sandwich. It was a little gritty, but I ate it—using it as a springboard for a lecture on trace elements in our diet.

Have you ever pulled a big, woody carrot out of the ground, rinsed it in the horse tank, and eaten it on the spot? It is actually quite sweet—very tasty, of course, but sweet! Gritty too! Your taste buds recognized the food value and rewarded you with the pleasures of flavors! Now, open a can of carrots, and compare. If it is sweet, read the label—flavors have been added. The canned product has been cleaned of all traces of soil. Even the outer layers have been brushed off, exposing the delicate enzyme systems. The life in the carrot drifts away long before you eat it. And so it is with all processed foods. Nutrients are lost or destroyed by simple exposure to each other. *Enzyme systems self-destruct when the protective cell structure is altered.*

Soil may have been a vital part of our diet in the past; iron, copper, zinc, manganese, cobalt, molybdenum, iodine, fluoride, bromine, selenium, chromium, vanadium nickel, lithium, cadmium, and many other soil elements have been shown to have biochemical roles in our bodies. Of course, since they are in soil, they get into vegetables (and animal foods) through the food chain. But there was much more soil in our food in the past, and it probably played a dietary role.

Why do so many people feel refreshed and invigorated after camping out? Is it simply the fresh air and exercise? Or did the plain old supermarket food take on a new nutritional dimension when dirt and soot were added at the camp site? Soil micronutrient enrichment? Just a thought! It can't be ruled out.

Symptoms of Micronutrient Deficiency

Experimenters learn which trace elements are needed by intentionally depriving their experimental animals of whatever element they're studying. Animals have been placed on diets lacking many things. I have just glanced over the list of some problems that can appear:

Copper deficiency in lambs and pigs can cause aortic aneurysm, which is a weakened bulge in a large artery.

Zinc deficiency can cause irritability and loss of hair. It plays an important role in protein metabolism, and I have heard of humans using zinc to help repair sore knee cartilage. Without zinc, lead comes to the fore, to cause such things as male impotence.

Manganese-deficient guinea pigs had diabetes. It cleared when the element was replaced in their diet.

Fluoride deficiency caused cavities in humans.

Chromium deficiency gives rats diabetes.

Cadmium levels may be related to high blood pressure in humans.

The importance of some elements is widely recognized: iodine for human thyroid metabolism. Low iodine levels in some areas of the world cause severe problems. In the Andes regions of Ecuador, the iodine was so low that about half the population suffered from *goiter* (an enlarged thyroid gland in the neck) or *cretinism* (a form of mental retardation when children are born with low thyroid function). Iodine is rich in ocean water and can be found in seafoods. It is also carried by the wind to coastal soils where it reaches the food chain. However, mountains prevent iodine from reaching the soil in many inland areas. The soil is low in iodine; so iodized salt has been introduced to prevent the deficiency diseases.*

Cobalt and iron are needed in blood formation. Cobalt is in vitamin B_{12} and iron is widely accessible. Cobalt can be found in buckwheat, figs, cabbage, lettuce, spinach, beet greens, and watercress. Liver is a good food source for both iron and cobalt. Actually, liver, because of its rich content of enzymes, is a good source for manganese, molybdenum, chromium, selenium and other metals; the metals are a vital part of enzyme molecules. For that reason, I think we all should consider a dish of liver and onions as a possible source of micronutrients *whenever a vague craving appears.* If it is a metal that is needed, liver probably contains it! Egg yolk is rich in phosphorous, iron, and copper. Seafood is rich in iodine and fluorine.

How Much Micronutrient?

If something is present as one part in a million parts of water, it is reported as 1 ppm. Fluoride prevents most cavities at a concentration of 1 ppm; but it causes ugly mottled teeth at 14 ppm.

When the dilution is one part in a billion parts of water, it is called 1 ppb. Drinking water in the United States varies in its iodine content from 0.01 to 73.3 ppb. Low levels are associated with the serious problems of low thyroid function (goiter and mental retardation).

Fluoride is added to drinking water in some areas to bring the level up to the "protective level." Iodine is added to table salt to be used in areas low in that element.

We need about a milligram of fluoride each day. If drinking

---

* Some orthomolecular specialists claim it's OK to salt your food with iodized salt on the grounds that it's the best way to get iodine in the diet. I feel the disadvantages of salt in masking your taste and influencing blood pressure far outweigh the chance of being low in iodine. Seafood is plentiful just about everywhere in this country.

water has 1 ppm, we need a million milligrams of water—or a thousand grams—or a liter (about a quart).

We need about 140 *micro*grams (millionths of a gram) of iodine each day. If drinking water contains 70 ppb, we need two billion micrograms of water—or two million milligrams or two thousand grams—or two liters (a little more than two quarts). If you can't get seafood you *can* drink water!

Get Your Nutrients in Whole Foods

Some people use bone meal for minerals. I worry about the calcium load in the kidneys, and stick to whole milk for my calcium salts.

Others take a one-a-day vitamin with minerals. I just don't have that much faith in the vitamin industry. Iron, zinc, and other minerals come in the right proportions in living things. And they have the micronutrients that are missing in pills. If you don't cook the minerals out of your food, they don't have to be added as a supplement!

One use of bone meal is with vitamin D to prevent the softening of the bones associated with menopause. This softening, called *osteoporosis,* is now known to be preventable with a simple exercise program—walking or jogging—that regularly increases the distance you can cover on foot. Adding bone meal with vitamin D is just an expensive way to get what a glass of whole milk has.

What about iron pills? I wouldn't have them in the house, as I've said: too dangerous. Try getting your iron from a little red meat, a whole egg, some green vegetables. In these food sources, you know that the iron is biologically available. (You can't trust a pill!)

If seeds, nuts, and eggs came with labels, we would all know that they are good sources for minerals! Just imagine what those labels would contain. And consider this: we probably don't know half of the good things that should be on a complete nutrient label of living things. This is why food is always the best way to get vitamins, and any other nutrients.

While we're on the subject of megavitamins and micronutrients, I should mention the common practice of using wheat-germ oil for endurance. The logic is in assuring high intake of EFAs and antioxidants (vitamin E) for use as fuel in long-distance events. While it is true that one of the EFAs (linoleic acid) has been identified as a primary source of energy beyond the thirty-kilometer mark, the amount in a normal mixed diet should be quite adequate.

The reason I have reservations about *regular* use of any oil is the effect of oil on the mean life expectancy of experimental mice. Oils rich in EFAs have been used to protect humans and animals from atherosclerosis; however, the choice in these studies was between EFAs and a diet *deficient* in EFAs. Mice lived the longest when they were fed a normal mixed chow of whole foods. When 20 percent lard was added, they had a shortened life expectancy; but when safflower oil high in EFAs was substituted as 20 percent of the diet, they did not live as long as those on lard! Antioxidants were added to the safflower diet, and the mice lived longer—*but not as long as the mice on the normal mixed diet of whole food!*

Therefore, I try to eat a mixed diet of whole foods, and am afraid of oils, which are extracted from something. Extraction is a form of processing; and I am afraid that an essential nutrient will *always* be lost in processing.

For example, take an ordinary egg. Egg yolk, without the protein in the white, can cause atherosclerosis in animals. By the same token, raw egg white, without the biotin in the yolk, can cause "egg-white injury" in animals and humans. Raw egg white removes biotin from the diet and causes nausea, skin eruptions, muscle pains, and depression. This condition can be treated with egg yolks. It does not occur with *cooked* egg white.

Whole egg does not cause disease! Separating yolk from white is a form of processing—which can be fatal to lab animals!

Take whole milk as another example. Butterfat, without the milk protein, can cause atherosclerosis in pigs. Whole milk does not. In fact, whole milk *lowers* the cholesterol in humans drinking four quarts a day!

Back to wheat-germ oil. It contains a wonderful list of EFAs and can be used to raise your tissue levels of EFAs. Short periods of use can help you lose weight when combined with a vigorous exercise program. However, you must be aware of the mouse experiments and worry about the excess intake of lipid oxides. Keep the oil fresh, in small dark bottles in the refrigerator. Taste it carefully. If it tastes rancid, dump it out!

Living seeds like sunflower seed come with a huge store of EFAs and vitamin E. So does living wheat grain. Grind your wheat the day you bake, and you will have ample EFAs.

When you are trying to lose weight, it is important to keep your diet rich in EFAs. The EFAs are needed when you try to burn stored body fat, which is usually very saturated.

If an athlete tells me that wheat-germ oil gives him endurance, then I know that his past diet has been very saturated—lots of animal products, especially steaks. Football players who turn to long-distance running will find wheat-germ oil helps them lose weight and run longer distances. However, after they have adopted the marathon runner's diet, the oils will have less noticeable benefit, because the diet comes with adequate EFAs. That is my point: Oils rich in EFAs help only if the diet has been deficient in EFAs. Once the basic needs are met with whole foods, the extra oils have no benefit—and much possible hazard from the surplus of toxic lipid oxides.

My concern over the hazards of oils extends to liquid shortenings. That is why I prefer my bread made with whole milk (with its natural butterfat) instead of water plus oils that have been processed in some way. Bread is OK *without* fat, too.

VITAMINS AND MINERALS IN A NUTSHELL (OR AN EGGSHELL, OR A KERNEL!)

I started this chapter by telling you all the possible bad things that can happen with vitamins—megadoses of them. You might have thought I was building a case against them. Now you see that the good things about them are dazzling compared to the few dangers: A, D, and iron aren't needed in pill form.

My second point was that the beneficial aspects of *large doses* of vitamins are well documented in the world's leading laboratories. B complex, C, and E are especially important, again, in large doses. Yet, as nutritionist George Briggs and all the rest who are responsible for the government's "Recommended Daily Allowance" keep saying, the vast majority of doctors feel that a balanced diet supplies all we need. The orthomolecularists, led by Linus Pauling, Carl C. Pfeiffer, and Abram Hoffer, counter with the obvious question: all we *need* for the absence of sickness or for the fullness of health?

Pauling points out that vitamin C may have been necessary for man in great quantities in prehistoric evolutions. Something happened, and now man can't synthesize the C he needs. So he commonly comes down with colds, heart disease, cancer . . . Most of the studies that tend to discredit the effect of vitamins, especially C, are useless because they involve small doses! So the question isn't: Vitamins, yes or no? The question is: Vitamins, how much? If you have any confidence in scientific studies, you will answer, along with me: *Large vitamin supplements for the full flush of health and long-term protection against disease.*

My third point is that the best way to get the large doses of vitamins you need, in the quantities best for you, is to eat the foods your body craves. Your cravings won't lie to you *if*—a big if—you have not disguised your real cravings with a salt-heavy, sugar-heavy, fat-heavy, no-exercise style of life.

Don't be fooled by the claim so often made that the vitamins and minerals in pills are chemically the same as those in foods. "Your body can't tell the difference," these pseudo-scientists say. There are four things wrong with this gross simplification. First, there is always room for error, intentional or not, on the part of the pill manufacturer; nature doesn't make mistakes. Second, vitamins in foods are often more easily assimilated into the body; they're biologically more available. Third, vitamins and minerals in foods bring many other nutrients along to the party—how many, we may never know. Fourth, pills don't talk! No one ever craved a pill. Your food cravings are your built-in regulators of quantity and freshness. A stale pill won't tell you anything.

Another bit of misdirection is the current fad of exchanging one food for another, ostensibly because they both have the same C or E or mineral value. This practice comes from too many pills: we begin to treat food like pills. A newspaper nutritionist advises that a half-pint of yogurt has little more nutritive value than a glass of skim milk; conclusion: the milk is a "better buy." Perhaps—if the yogurt is gussied up with flavorings and sugar, as many brands are these days. But yogurt has a lot of things in it that skim milk doesn't. If your body craves yogurt, maybe it's trying to tell you it's not the calcium it wants, but the cultures.

Remember the "parsley principle." Food that's impractical to eat can't do you any good. Keeping food that wilts in your refrigerator because no one wants it is an expensive way to release your guilt feelings.

I don't mean to scare you away from a good diet by mentioning nutrition together with marathon races! The Whole Life Diet is for everyone, not just joggers and runners. If the post-cardiac patient can find an exercise level to open up the lines of communication between body and food, so can anyone. And the endurance event that's best for you will become your own laboratory of nutrition. It's another way of finding your bodyprint.

But, you say, the advocates of vitamins make far-reaching claims, not just for optimum health, but also for *healing*. If you've followed me this far, explore that fascinating world with me now!

EIGHT
Healing
with
Food

"Less than a year to live?"

Shultz and I were at the two-mile mark, running along Crest Road, waiting for the sun to come up.

"Gwen, my mother-in-law," repeated Shultz, "the doctors back East give her less than a year to live!"

I was starting to sweat, so I looked for a tree branch to hang my T-shirt on. I tried to reassure him that doctors were not always right about such things. After all, in my work I had seen thousands of cases of sudden death. No one can be that certain, either way!

He began to tell me about Gwen's medical problems—a familiar story for widows in their seventies. She was well taken care of by a devoted daughter, had her own room with TV. Meals and laundry were done. She saw her doctors about twice a month. The list of problems was endless: arthritis, diabetes, arteriosclerosis, hypertension, constipation, varicose veins, and on and on. Her shopping list contained over ten types of medicines. There were pills to control sugar in her urine, pain pills, water pills, salt pills, constipation pills, red pills, white pills, short and long capsules.

Her doctors began to lose hope when she had the small stroke that left her too weak to walk without help. She had a four-legged wooden "walker" to get around in her room. The arthritic pain required more and more medication. Her constipation also progressed each month—smaller, harder stools, more pain. Her feet swelled and a small ulcer appeared above her ankle. It did not heal. The ulcer turned green and the skin of her whole leg became hot and pink. Another pill, an antibiotic, was added.

Gwen had to see physicians about twice a week when the leg ulcer upset her diabetic control. An X ray of the leg showed that her bones were OK, but the pain really began to bother her. She couldn't tell if it was the pain of arthritis or inflammation.

I had to admit that Gwen was in trouble!

Shultz continued to press me. "You're a doctor," he said. "Tell me what to do!"

This would be the first patient I referred to Nathan Pritikin. I had met him through the Seniors Track Club, and had heard that he gave dietary advice to very sick people with some surprisingly good results. As Nathan's headquarters were then in Santa Barbara, he could be reached by phone each day. He consented to guide Gwen through her shopping and cooking activities only if she was under the care of a physician. An internist, "Big Ben," also of the same track club, consented to monitor Gwen's diabetic control and other problems. Pritikin isn't a physician, but he enjoys working through cooperative physicians in cases like this.

I have to admit I was skeptical, back in those days. I was certain that diet and exercise were important for health, of course; but I thought you had to start early in life to see benefits. I just did not have Nathan's optimism.

Gwen arrived by plane, looking much sicker than I had expected. Nathan had specific instructions for the *first meal* on the West Coast. No added fat! No simple sugars or salt! The meals required long shopping trips for whole foods—foods "as grown."

Over the phone he told her to walk as far as she could, eight
times a day, and write down the number of *steps!* Six steps was
a long walk. She was very weak, so he told her: "Don't hit the
furniture if you fall!"

Gwen was encouraged to do as much of the shopping and
cooking as she could, gradually taking over her own care. She
complained at first, but Nathan stressed to her that the exercise
was just as vital as the diet.

The leg ulcer was not where I expected. It was above the
ankle all right, but not on the side of the leg where varicose
ulcers occur. It was in front, over the shin bone.

"How did you get this?"

"I bumped it several weeks ago," Gwen explained. "But I
kept it covered up with stockings so my daughter wouldn't
worry."

"This is Southern California," I said. "Take it outside on the
patio—let's see—ten minutes, four times a day, in bright sun.
Keep it uncovered during the day. Air and sun should take care
of it."

She continued to walk from table to wall, wall to chair,
chair to chair, and finally to the door. Her total number of steps
increased each day.

I couldn't understand how diet would affect Gwen's condition. Her confusion cleared. She needed less pain medication
in a week, less diabetic medication in two weeks. Her blood-
pressure medication was no longer needed at the end of the
month. The ulcer on her leg cleared up. She forgot all about
constipation; her stools were huge and soft. In six weeks, she
went to have her hair done and bought a new dress. After three
months she hosted a dinner party at Shultz's house, and was
ready to fly back East to visit her other daughter. The diet had
worked!

THE PRITIKIN DIET

Nathan Pritikin is Director of the Longevity Research Institute
in Santa Monica, California. His diet evolved as a result of the
institute's own research into medical literature. It reflects the

"high fiber" ideas of Burkitt in England, the population studies of Trowell, and the observations on the effects of diet on health in many countries around the world. It is not strictly a vegetarian diet; about a pound and a half of lean meat, fish, or poultry is allowed each week. It is a diet very similar to that of the Tarahumara Indians and other primitive peoples.

Nathan's diet is very low in fat—only 10 percent of the total—and all the fat comes as intrinsic parts of the food. No fat can be added!

The 10 percent fat diet has been used to reverse atherosclerosis in animals, and it lowers the blood fats so dramatically that the oxygen-carrying capacity of the blood increases in just a few days. This would help explain Gwen's improved concentration. Her confusion cleared quickly.

Of course all the work she had to do, preparing the meals and shopping, kept her busy burning calories. Soup, for example, was made all from whole ingredients. A trip to the supermarket involved picking up white turnips, yellow turnips, onions, celery, carrots, green pepper, zucchini, green beans, squash, and tomato paste. The afternoon would be spent chopping all this. When cooking was going on she had to add salsa, garlic powder, onion powder, cumin, and oregano.

She complained about the hard work—but she improved.

Nathan's diet is purposely very high in fiber. Cereal bran is put on salads, on hot cereal, in soup, and in bread. The fiber cured the constipation, of course, but it also prevented the absorption of much of the salt in the gut—lowering the blood pressure.

The fiber contained silicon—reducing arthritic pains and eliminating the need for pain pills.

Her diabetes came under control as her diet took effect. Complex carbohydrates—starches—are absorbed slowly from the gut all day. The blood sugar doesn't get a chance to rise when exercise balances caloric intake. No matter how much Gwen ate, she couldn't gain weight—the vegetables in the diet contained only 200 calories per pound! Soups, salads, and snacks that added up to four pounds per day would carry only 800 calories! Small amounts of meat, fruit, and bread were also used; but the meat was lean and the fruit was limited because of the simple sugars they contained.

"Big Ben," Gwen's doctor, did all the usual blood tests and gave her an exercise test to make certain she was OK. He was happy to stop the pills when the diet made them unnecessary.

Gwen continued to improve as her shopping and cooking ability returned. It had been years since she took care of herself. When she flew back East, she needed only an occasional pill for her diabetes. Her walking mileage added up to three or four miles each day! I began to wonder why more people weren't eating like this!

Gwen's Typical Day—Eight Meals

Cereal: 4 oz cracked wheat, cooked, with 4 oz of skim milk and a half a banana add up to 200 calories. The shopping list for cereals included oatmeal and brown rice also—variety!

Fruit #1: Fresh raw fruit is limited to four pieces per day— whole oranges, pears, apples, grapes. The morning "fruit break" was usually a whole grapefruit, for 100 calories.

Salad: A giant 1½-lb salad contains only 150 calories. Gwen would take half a pound of lettuce for a base and add sliced raw carrots, tomatoes, sprouts, cucumbers, radishes, chayote, celery, and broccoli until the salad weighed 1½ lbs. The dressing consisted of cider vinegar, lemon juice, and apple juice, with the appropriate spices—blended onion power, garlic powder, paprika, dried parsley, dry mustard, and oregano.

Soup #1: An 8-oz crunchy soup, using large pieces of chopped vegetables: 50 calories.

Potato: A baked potato with tomato soup added instead of butter; chopped onions, tomato, and sprouts add character. No salt or oils are allowed on this diet. About 150 calories for a half-pound potato.

Soup #2: Gwen ran vegetables through a blender and cooked with brown rice, adding chili powder, garlic powder, and oregano to taste. An 8-oz serving was 50 calories.

Dinner: One pound of vegetables containing tiny scraps of chicken, stir-fried with fat-free broth. About 200 calories. The vegetables included bok choy (Chinese cabbage), Chinese pea pods, mushrooms, green peppers, onions, and celery. Soy sauce, water chestnuts, and bamboo shoots added flavor and color.

Fruit #2: The eighth meal is a bedtime snack of raw fruit— another 100 calories.

Supplement: If more than 1,000 calories are needed, whole-wheat bread (with no salt or shortening), or 4 oz of brown rice is added to dinner.

Since Gwen's successful experience, I have seen many others try the Pritikin diet with similar results. The patients who can bring themselves to stop smoking and start walking find the diet works for them. Pritikin has put many of his recipes into a cook-book. However, if you take any of your favorite recipes and remove all fat, salt, and simple sugars, you will probably have a pretty safe food. The diet is supposed to be 10 percent fat, 15 percent protein, and 75 percent carbohydrates. Most of the carbohydrates are complex starch in vegetables and grains.

Here's Why the Pritikin Diet Works

By now, many of the nutritional principles involved in the Pritikin diet are familiar to you. Let's see how they work in cases like Gwen's:

Atherosclerosis: This disease of narrowed arteries can be improved in animals by feeding them a diet that is only 10 per-cent fat. A high-fiber diet also helps remove the fatty deposits in the arteries of animals. Humans with chest pain (angina) or leg pains (claudication) also improve clinically. They have fewer symptoms almost as soon as the blood fat drops. The exercise helps them burn up unwanted fat; and, when they stop smoking, blood cells are available to carry oxygen.

Arthritis: Gout improves if you reduce your intake of animal protein. Other types of arthritis improve when fiber intake in-creases, because of the extra silicon in the fiber. Two pounds of raw vegetables and fruit contain over 1,000 milligrams of vitamin C, and this can help both arthritis and atherosclerosis.

Diabetes: Exercise and a high fiber intake will lower your blood sugar and help control diabetes. Starchy foods are much better for a diabetic than a high-fat diet or simple sugars.

High Blood Pressure: Exercise, fiber, and a low-salt diet bring the blood pressure down. The raw fruits and vegetables have less sodium than potassium. This is more natural.

Obesity: No one can put on weight eating food as grown. Since most of the permitted foods average less than 200 calories per pound, it is impossible to eat more than you need. The extra exercise burns off calories—and you lose weight.

Constipation, etc.: It has been said that eating five pounds of vegetables a day will cause you to gain three pounds a day for three days; then you have a nine-pound bowel movement! This is not true, of course. You do feel as if you are gaining weight, eating all day long; but the scales will show no change. Your body is getting rid of the extra salt and fat it had stored. Then by the end of the week, your gut is adjusting to the frequent small meals. Your stools are much larger than you have ever seen, of course, but they amount only to about a pound a day—mostly fiber and water. Without small, hard stools, you cannot be constipated. Also, you cannot get appendicitis, hemorrhoids, hiatal hernia, gallbladder trouble, or diverticulitis. All of these conditions require small, hard stools—impossible on the Pritikin diet.

Why Isn't Everyone on the Diet?

It *is* a lot of work. You can't eat TV dinners. You can't go to your favorite fast-food place. You must do a lot of walking in supermarkets and then a lot of chopping at home. For some meals, you must start a day ahead—soaking hard beans or cooling a fatty stew in the refrigerator so you can skim off the fat.

Someone must work in the kitchen: baking bread, sprouting grain, playing with spices. Eight small meals a day means that there is always a dish to be washed.

Exercise isn't much fun alone. If you're the only one in your neighborhood who wants to go for a walk, it can be lonely out there, especially if the weather is bad.

Breaking old habits is hard. If you have smoked for twenty or thirty years, it is hard to give it up—even for medical reasons.

Even if you think you are on the Pritikin diet, there is

always doubt. Did someone put shortening in your bread? Is this can of vegetables really free from salt? It's a lot of work if you are doing it by yourself. That is why Pritikin encourages the spouse or roommate to attend the diet conferences to learn the lifestyle with the patient.

WHEN DIETING NEEDS A
DOCTOR'S SUPERVISION

When you elect to follow a strict diet, such as the Pritikin diet, you should be under a doctor's care in the following situations:

Medications: Suppose you're taking medications for diabetes, gout, hypertension, and atherosclerosis (angina-like chest pain, or the leg cramps of claudication). You should let your doctor know that you are trying to substitute mileage for medication, and that you are going to need less medication as your habits of eating and exercise improve. Your goal is to be able to get along without any medication, eventually! However, you should be working with a doctor who believes in exercise and diet, so he will be ready to reduce your prescriptions as the need for them decreases. It's dangerous to take these drugs when they are no longer needed!

High Blood Pressure: If you are taking pills to control your blood pressure, you can buy a blood-pressure cuff and follow your blood pressure at home—take it twice in both arms twice a day until you get bored taking it. Then you'll get a relaxed reading. Increase food fiber until your stool floats; and increase walking mileage until you are doing six miles a day. Use no salt.

Usually, after four weeks of floating stools, and six miles a day, blood pressure will be normal without pills!

Diabetes: Follow the levels of sugar in your urine with tests at home. Your doctor can teach you how to test it easily with a simple paper strip. Increase your mileage to six miles a day, walking—keeping in mind that exercise calories do not require insulin. Eat whole foods, as grown, and avoid simple sugars. The *simple* sugars like table sugar, brown sugar, honey, and molasses are absorbed too fast and spill into the urine. (See Chapter Four for the glucose-insulin trap.) Starchy calories are absorbed slowly all day. About half the diabetics on this regimen have been able to stop medication without spilling sugar into their urine. Almost all patients have greatly reduced their use of drugs for controlling diabetes.

Heart Disease: Chest pain or leg pain due to narrowed arteries can also improve, but only your doctor can tell you how *fast* you can safely go. He doesn't know how *far;* that depends on many other factors: weather, diet, clothing, and sense of humor. If your doctor has taught you to take your pulse, you can exercise with relative safety—you'll be as safe walking as sitting in front of the TV set! Your doctor should be involved in these exercise programs, so he can guide you and his other patients into greater and greater distances. If he walks or runs also, he can tell you about stretching, diet, shoes, injuries, and so forth.

There's nothing wrong with a doctor prescribing drugs *if* he educates the patient at the same time. Your urine sugar, blood pressure, and exercise pulse rate are *your* responsibility as well as your doctor's. His use of pills should be considered temporary. Your corrected diet and exercise habits should correct the problem, making pills unnecessary. But *you* must know when to stop the pills.

Physician-educators can reach large numbers of patients at the same time when they help out the local YMCA exercise classes. The Central YMCA in Honolulu has had a class for cardiac patients for many years. They also conduct classes in Kapiolani Park with the help of Honolulu's Department of Parks and Recreation—again reaching large numbers of interested citizens at the same time. If they have a two-hour fun run, thousands of people come, and afterward they hold a huge picnic. I have met many patients in these programs in Honolulu. They all understand their disease very well; and they know when medication is important and when it is dangerous. That's what I call "preventive medicine"—the use of mileage and diet, rather than medications!

AND NOW FOR SOME LESS FATAL
BUT MORE ANNOYING
PROBLEMS . . .

Hemorrhoids and Constipation

You cannot have symptoms of hemorrhoids unless your stools are small and hard. Actually, the "hemorrhoids" are natural veins and serve a useful purpose of helping control the time you pass your stools. They have special glands and nerves that enable you to time your bowel movements for socially acceptable times. You damage these structures when you try to pass a hard stool; and the damage causes the swelling, inflammation, and pain. If you are on a high-fiber diet, you pass large, soft stool; and the hemorrhoidal veins serve a normal function—and do not become damaged every time you have a bowel movement. Soft stool also prevents appendicitis, diverticulitis, hiatal hernia, varicose veins, and a variety of other ailments.

You can allow the hemorrhoids to heal if you get on a high-fiber diet; the "cure" is almost miraculous! One cup of raw bran, boiled, and spread over three or four meals, will keep stools soft. (Do not take a cup of bran without first boiling it; just add boiling water to a quarter-cup four times a day, and soak five minutes.)

But start cereal bran intake gradually! If you are not on a high-fiber diet, your transit time is three days—in other words, you have three days' food supply in your gut. If you add a cup of bran a day to your diet, your transit time is reduced to one day; you carry a meal around only one day before it is passed! The danger of starting too fast is clear if you imagine that two thirds of your food is trying to take three days to travel through you and then along comes one third of your gut traveling the same distance in one day! With the fast transit-time food in back, there is a good chance that you'll have severe cramps and diarrhea. However, if you gradually increase the fiber in your diet, you can adjust slowly to the fast transit time—and cure your hemorrhoidal symptoms.

Once you are on a high-fiber diet with fast transit times you might ask about the hazards of carrying around stool for three days when only one will do. Constipated individuals do carry around small, hard stool in their colon. *It is this extra time that stool uses to break down molecules and form carcinogens.*. High-fiber diets are associated with low numbers of colon cancers in population studies; and I like to think that preventing hemorrhoids with bran also prevents *cancer* of the large bowel. So fiber, like vitamins E and C, is associated with some "protection" against cancer.

My Knee Hurts. What Do I Do?

Check your bad habits. Do your stools float? If not, your intake of *silicon* is too low. Add full-fiber foods to your diet and avoid "refined" foods and "empty calories." Drink alfalfa tea; put dry alfalfa leaves in your soup, meatloaf, salads, etc. Grind alfalfa leaves with your oats in your coffee-bean grinder and add the resultant "green flour" to your daily Super Drink. (If you don't know what a Super Drink is, make one up of your own, using milk, raw egg, malt, fruit, wheat germ, ice cream, yeast flakes, and yogurt—aiming for the consistency of eggnog or a milk shake.)

If your stools float, next check your intake of vitamin C. Are you averaging a gram of ascorbic acid or sodium ascorbate for each ten kilometers?

Your knee is a good index of all your bad habits. If you think your diet is adequate, then your knee shouldn't hurt. If your knee does hurt, look first at your diet!

CRAVINGS: YOUR BODY IS TRYING TO TELL YOU SOMETHING

Almost everyone who is put on a strict diet gets the urge to cheat, sooner or later. Old cravings come back, and extra salt, fat, or sugar is eaten. Why do they cheat?

If you're put on a diet, it's important to stick to it when your disease prevents you from doing your six miles a day. It's important when you still need medication for an underlying condition. However, after you no longer need medication, and while you are doing your six miles a day, the diet can be relaxed a bit. Pritikin allows for this by having both a strict "reversal" diet and a more relaxed "maintenance" diet.

Cravings for things not on the diet are important, and most people eventually obey their cravings. I think there's a biological reason for cravings, and I encourage you to analyze any strong desire you have to eat certain foods. Why do you want to eat that? What is it you really want? Your body is trying to tell you something; are you getting the message straight?

Cravings are always possible when you are following a rigid diet designed by someone who is not in your kitchen. Industry may alter something, and a micronutrient may vanish or a new contaminant might appear. Eating food as grown is safest when the cook is also designing the menu. Grandmother tasted as she prepared meals. Her cravings altered eating habits, guiding the family's nutrition. If she craved things with ascorbic acid, heaps of green leafy vegetables appeared on the supper table. If she craved an amino acid, eggs or meat became a prominent part of the meal. So it was, I suppose, with the minerals. Blackstrap molasses was conspicuous when iron or another mineral was required.

Tom Jones, a powerful marathoner in my neighborhood, had a grandmother in Denmark who did all her cooking with potato water. She swore that it gave her family strength! (It gave them vitamin C, among other things.) Her idea of "bread" was a heavy, dark bread containing many different foods: potatoes, honey, molasses, cornmeal, rye flour, whole-wheat flour, and caraway seeds. An egg was smeared on the top to give it a crust to stick more seeds into; whole milk was used instead of lard for the shortening. She called it whole-wheat bread, but we know it as real old-fashioned pumpernickel. She called American bread "cake"—and she was right. Our soft white bread is a poor substitute for the type of bread our ancestors ate. Just review the ingredients she used; imagine the vital nutrients it would contain if it were made with freshly ground grains; corn, rye, wheat! *Her bread was designed by cravings; our bread was designed by industry.* Virtually all nourishment is omitted from ours.

Unfortunately, missing nourishment isn't the only problem with processed foods. Their flavors are distorted by sugar, salt, and other additives; and that leads to distorted, falsified cravings. But our instinctive cravings are there to tell us what nutrients we need, and we *can* learn to listen intelligently to our bodies. Using our cravings as a guide, and relying on whole foods to satisfy them, we should be able to meet our needs for nutrients.

Let's analyze some of the more common cravings, and see how to tell if the craving is honest or distorted.

Salt

Our taste buds can reward us with the pleasant flavor of "salt" when our bodies need *sodium*. If you are not taking medication and are running over six miles a day with normal blood pressure, then adding a pinch of salt to a baked potato or a bowl of soup can't hurt. If you are walking less than six miles a day, and have recently been on blood-pressure medication, then salt can be dangerous.

First, review your diet. Your tongue can't tell the difference between sodium and potassium. If the *potassium* has been leached out of foods by cooking, you may crave "salt" but not need the sodium molecule. Try eating raw fruits and vegetables. Increase your *water* intake to see if the salt craving is simply thirst.

If your salt craving is just taste-bud boredom, use hot chili peppers, garlic, onions, thyme, and other herbs to *spice* up the meal.

If you tried eating a raw diet with lots of spices and the salt cravings persist, use a little salt and check your blood pressure. This is especially important if salt cravings are associated with weakness. If your blood pressure isn't high, salt is OK.

Sugar

Cavemen found very few sweets in the woods. Honey was defended by bees. Fruits ripened once a year. Chewing whole grain for the trace of starch sweetness was probably their most common way of handling their craving for sweets. Now, of course, we can fill our kitchen with pounds of refined sugar, and put it in every dish with disastrous results. That is not normal!

However, a strict diet of only complex carbohydrate (without simple sugars) may seem too severe to you. If you are tempted to cheat and eat a sweet, analyze your cravings. If you are not a diabetic, and you have just finished a six-mile run, your intake of sweets probably has no significance. A dab of honey on your hot, whole-grain cereal is OK. Try cooking your oats with raisins for sweetness. Add chopped dates to bread dough. Raw fruit can make a cake out of simple whole-wheat dough.

If you are a mild diabetic patient who has reached the six-mile walk, a more cautious intake of simple sugar is wise. Check your urine for sugar whenever you "cheat" with simple sugars. Once your distance exceeds a twelve-mile walk once a week, you will probably *not* spill sugar into your urine when you increase your intake of natural sweets—fruits, dried fruit, honey, or molasses.

Unfortunately, I must still be concerned about sucrose. It produces disease so easily in animals that I suspect there may be some problems with trace elements or microcontamination in processed table sugar.

Fat

A high-fat diet can kill, as I've said—especially if it's unfriendly fat like burned cholesterol in steaks or abnormal *trans*-fat in hydrogenated vegetable oils like margarine or shortening.

If you think you crave fat, analyze the craving. What do you really want? No one can crave *grease*, for example. The deep-fried and breaded piece of fast food that looks so good to you has no food value. Your taste buds are telling you to eat it for reasons that are unrelated to the semiprocessed item itself. Think! Is it the *salt* you want? Is it the *starch* in the crust? Is it the *protein* inside the chicken, fish, or shrimp? *Deep-fried foods contain too many lipid oxides to be considered safe for human consumption.* Lipid oxides cause atherosclerosis in animals even when the animals are getting adequate fiber, essential fatty acids, and vitamins C and E. Try to satisfy the craving with something else.

Eggs have some fat and cholesterol. However, *whole* egg does not cause disease in well-nourished animals; and one egg per day did not raise human blood cholesterol in the tests we reviewed in Chapter Six. The egg may satisfy your cravings for deep-fried foods, if it was the protein or the fat you wanted. Poach the egg; avoid grease!

If you are a former cardiac patient, a safe formula for egg intake is "one egg for each six miles." There is *no* safe formula for grease or burned cholesterol in charbroiled steak!

Whole milk is another source of safe fat. Use it as a drink, or, when baking bread, substitute it for the water and shortening in the recipe.

If you cannot cover six miles on foot, it is wise to keep your fat intake to 10 percent of calories until you can. This usually takes only a few weeks in a supervised walking program.

Protein

If you crave a steak, and try to justify it on a need for protein, you are wrong! American steak, fattened in a feed lot with old grain, is high in saturated fat. Old grain is too low in EFAs these days, so beef tallow and hog lard are now more saturated than they were in grandmother's time. The modern steak is probably 60 percent *fat*, a very poor source of protein. Usable protein in whole-wheat bread comes very close to beef if the bread contains milk. Whole egg also matches beef nicely. Nuts, seeds, and whole grain contain biologically sound amounts of protein and fat—friendly fat—and can be increased to match your cravings for steak.

If you think that the steak may contain a micronutrient, use it to make soup. Refrigerate the soup to skim off the fat—and then reheat, adding crisp vegetables and brown rice. Beef muscle is a good source for carnitine (a B vitamin), iron, zinc, and other nutrients. However, this "refrigerator soup" has no fat!

If you must "cheat" on any diet, do it logically. Follow cravings that are likely to increase your ability to exercise. If something makes you feel stronger—eat it. You may want to try a beer for each six miles; an egg for each six miles; raw nuts and seeds each day; extra vitamin C or E. If the craving is associated with weakness, flush your face with a high-thiamin series of yeast, yogurt, and wheat germ. (See Chapter Seven.) As the high intake of thiamin flushes your face, it will also saturate your body's enzyme systems—giving you strength at the molecular level.

Nonspecific Cravings

These are the hardest to explain. As you learned in Chapter Seven, there are dozens of chemical elements in the earth's crust that play a role in biological life at concentrations so low that they were identified only recently. More will be discovered in the future. If your diet lacks some element from the soil that should be present in parts per million or parts per *billion*, then you are going to have to go camping and get a little soil in your food. Backpack for a day, even if it is only a mile into the park, and fix a meal over a fire outdoors. The wind will put some ashes and dust in your food. Carry a handbook of edible wild foods, and see if you can locate some of them. Putting a few wild dandelion leaves into your salad can't hurt, and it might help you put the subject of your own nutrition back into perspective. Backpacking combines mileage with meals—since you carry what you will eat. Former patients can appreciate their newfound fitness when it is expressed in terms of "kilometers hiked carrying a backpack"!

All right. People look at you kind of funny if you talk about putting a little ashes and dust in your food. But what flour mills do to grain is the real joke!

Why Take a One-a-Day Pill?

I like to think in terms of *results*. We all have been guilty of trusting the drug industry to provide us with a pill for nutritional insurance; but what are the results? Are we really preventing a deficiency, providing nutrition, or gaining pep and energy? Think!

If you need iron, eat a little liver and onions, an egg, some green vegetables, or whole grain. The advantage of this approach is the rich source of copper, zinc, and other metals that may never be put in a pill in *biologically meaningful* amounts.

If you think a pill can give you pep, compare the results of a "thiamin flush"—brought on by yeast, yogurt, and wheat germ—with a vitamin pill. Compare your energy level after a backpacking meal with a vitamin pill. Think!

Reading labels doesn't help much. Processed foods can have selected vitamins and minerals added to *sell* the package. However, I think there is a real difference between nourishing food and synthetic food with a few nutrients added. Whole foods do not come with printed labels, but you can look at them and see that they are alive. You can't see any evidence of life in a vitamin pill—or a box of processed food. Life is the key; eat living things! The vitamin industry has tried to "educate" us to think about the "chemistry of life." We can forget about chemistry if we concentrate on *life,* and try to eat living things. Living things contain things helpful to life that chemists have not yet dreamed of!

PODIATRISTS OR NUTRITION?

Orthotics are personalized structures placed in your shoes by a podiatrist to improve the way your foot strikes the ground. Usually a walker or a runner goes to a podiatrist for orthotics after pain has hampered his mileage.

You take your pain and your shoes to the podiatrist. Sounds logical, but I have a word of advice.

First, talk to someone your age who is already doing what you want to do—whether it is walking or running. There are people who have succeeded where you failed. They may find that you are doing a dumb thing like wearing the wrong shoes: too light to support you, too tight, or too worn out. It's a waste of time and money to find a podiatrist, buy orthotics, and then learn that you are doing a dumb thing!

If you have tried several good shoes and still have pain, it is time to sit down and think of the next thing you may be doing wrong—omitting the stretch. Experienced (and successful) walkers and runners have routines they follow to keep their muscles balanced. A simple sit-up, one for each mile, may be all that you need. You must learn these under supervision, so you get them right; and you must always avoid "overstretch," which is painful and can be dangerous. Enthusiasm is dangerous during your stretching and warm-up exercises. And remember that *time* during a stretch is more important than movement. Most muscles don't respond to stretching unless a position is held for thirty seconds or more.

If you are having pain in a joint or tendon, and you have tried new shoes and a variety of stretching and yoga exercises, it is still not time to try the podiatrist. Look at your diet. If your body can't handle protein well, joint cartilage and tendons will have weak protein—and mileage can hurt. Try an egg for each six miles. Take a zinc supplement for a while.

Alcoholics are turning to jogging as a substitute addiction for their drinking problems. Unfortunately, they may have liver damage already, and with weak livers, they will not be able to make good protein to hold together the joints during jogging. "Drinker's knee," as we have seen, is a common problem—pain in the knee after jogging. I tell such patients to stick to walking for a while. They can try increasing their intake of brewer's yeast, egg, milk, whole grain, lean meat, and other sources of natural vitamins and amino acids. However, I do not advise a "high-protein" diet. The water-soluble vitamins in the B-complex group are probably the most important. So if you have been drinking heavily, don't run to a podiatrist at the first sign of leg pains.

Cardiac patients may be low in silicon if their stools do not float. This indicates a low fiber intake. They may also be low in vitamin C. I tell them to take a gram of vitamin C for each six miles; and to increase their dietary fiber until their stools float. It takes about six weeks to load the body with silicon, as we have seen in the previous chapter. Low silicon levels will also result in leg and joint pains; again, don't assume it's time for the podiatrist!

Smokers also can use jogging as a substitute addiction and stop smoking when they reach the six-miles-a-day ability level. However, smokers have very low vitamin C levels in their tissues. Therefore, they often are stopped by knee pain before they reach the six-mile distance—"smoker's knee"! Again, they must remove the oxidant (tobacco smoke) and add the antioxidants (vitamin C and vitamin E) before the knee can heal.

Orthotics may help *the alcoholic cardiac patient who smokes,* but there are sound biochemical reasons why they will not. We all can benefit from some improvement in the way our feet strike the ground, but we can benefit only *if* our body chemistry *allows* us to make good cartilage and tendon tissue.

Questions to Ask Before You See a Podiatrist

1. Do I have the proper shoes, and are they in good repair?
2. Have I been doing my stretching exercises properly?
3. Do my stools float?
4. Am I getting a gram of ascorbic acid for each six miles?
5. Am I avoiding tobacco smoke and distilled alcohol?
6. Is my diet adequate in protein?
7. Have I waited six weeks after correcting any of the above?
8. Have I consulted a more experienced runner?
9. Have I read a book written by a *running* podiatrist?

Dose Anyone *Really* Need Orthotics?

Certainly! Nature didn't design us all to be joggers and runners. Some feet are so bad that they need some help even for hiking long distances. However, not everyone needs orthotics. Everyone *does* need good nutrition; and, until you correct your nutritional deficiencies, you will have trouble with long mileage.

Some running podiatrists have written some good books with whole chapters on what to do instead of going to the podiatrist's office. One of my running friends, John Pagliano of Long Beach, California, starts his lectures with instructions for simple, do-it-yourself alterations to shoes to prevent foot problems from bringing runners into his office.

To summarize: there are good, sound reasons why food can heal even such seemingly mechanical problems as bad knees. But you must know what you're suffering from, what nutrients you're lacking, and how to get them into your diet. You must also learn to think for yourself about your body, and pay attention to what it's telling you.

NINE
Food Folklore

Folklore is the speculation of our ancestors. They didn't have scientific facts for a base, but they had generations of experience. What do we have now? A recent article in *Science* made the point that the Jewish mother's chicken soup has curative powers beyond custom and cultural expectation. Every day we're uncovering some scientific fact to corroborate an old wives' tale. Or is it simply hankering after the past, an "old-time" syndrome?

ANCIENT WISDOM

Whatever folklore may be, I think it's worth exploring in the context of a Whole Life Diet. If twenty million Frenchmen can't be wrong, I think it's a fair guess that twenty generations can't be too far off, either.

If, as I claim in this book, it's critical to trust our natural cravings, one would expect that over the centuries the cravings should have become solidified in some kind of theory. That's why I think we have a scientific basis for folklore: *cravings*. We don't need a Jung or a Freud to direct us: the centuries should have made their point.

Folklore: Werewolves Howl by the Light of the Full Moon

If anyone called upon me to do an autopsy on a werewolf, I'd certainly have a high level of skepticism. After all, the subject of werewolves is not covered in current medical texts. However, I can imagine the story from the witnesses would go something like this:

He runs howling through the woods. He used to look like a normal human being, but now he has the face and hands of a wolf—hairy brown skin, short, wide nose with exposed, flaring nostrils; bright red teeth exposed all the time. His hands are like paws—no fingers like a man's. We only see him like that when there's a full moon.

Ridiculous, you say? Probably not! There is a genetic defect that did exist in the populations where the werewolf stories appeared. This defect, called *congenital erythropoietic porphyria*, results in the clinical picture described above. The metabolic pathway for making blood pigment is defective, and abnormal pigments, called *porphyrins*, accumulate in the body tissues. Porphyrins give the teeth a bright red color, and make the skin very sensitive to sunlight. People with this disease cannot go out in the daylight; they prefer moonlight, becoming nocturnal.

Patients appear relatively normal at birth, but soon the hair grows out on the face to protect it from sunlight. Skin turns dark brown for the same reason. If sunlight does strike the skin, it causes severe pain and damage. The nose and eyelids can actually fall off. The face is so disfigured that the resemblance to a wolf may be striking. Fingers can fall off when the skin gets exposed to sun, ulcerates, and scars down; the resemblance to a wolf's paw is, again, striking. But most interesting is the severe pain that sends the patients running, "howling," around the room (or through the woods).

This explanation for the origins of the werewolf legend can

be found in the medical literature.[1] Of course, all physicians study porphyria in medical school; the condition has been reported in many countries. So if I did do such an autopsy, I would recognize the brilliant red teeth and realize that I was dealing with a real medical problem—not a legend.

Now, if werewolves can be explained in a logical, scientific way, what else can we learn from folklore? How many things have we rejected as tall tales, when they are really true? By the same token, are there things we accept as *fact*, when they should be considered mere *fantasy?*

I think there are—especially when it comes to the subject of nutrition. Take the remedy for porphyria. If carrots are eaten in huge numbers, the yellow pigment, carotene, colors the skin yellow—protecting it from sunlight. The person with porphyria can stay out in the sun five times longer protected this way.

Folklore: Garlic Keeps Vampires Away

Before the era of the local medical examiner, there was considerable folklore surrounding the subject of death. Why would the simple folk of a rural village make up a story about a horrifying night visitor? Obviously, they just misinterpreted what they saw. If a member of the family was jolly and alive at bedtime, but dead in the morning, the sudden death could be blamed on an evil force of some kind. This would be easy if the victim of sudden death carried a horrified expression of rigor mortis—appearing to have died in a struggle with the unseen night visitor. Often, there is a small amount of blood-tinged saliva that dries on the cheek and neck. Unless inspection was thorough, you could easily pass this off as a bite in the neck by a vampire.

Most of these sudden deaths were probably due to strokes or heart attacks. Statistically, garlic eaters would have fewer such deaths. Garlic removed atherosclerosis from rabbits while they were still eating the cholesterol.[2] As we have seen, garlic also protected humans from butter.[3] When they ate butter alone, serum cholesterol levels rose; but when they ate garlic with butter, they fell. Obviously, those who eat much garlic must have a lot in the kitchen—the protection against "vampires" would be obvious to all the neighbors and friends. (Onions also protected against butter; the ratio for 100 grams of butter is 50 grams onion or 25 grams garlic. That's Italian cooking!)

One of the molecules in garlic, called *allin*, has been isolated and found to inhibit both bacteria and tumor cells.[4] This could explain the variety of diseases garlic has been used for, dating back to Hippocrates, who prescribed it for pneumonia and infected wounds.

Folklore: An Apple a Day Keeps the Doctor Away

One apple contains enough silicon in the pectin to supply the whole day's requirement. The amount of vitamin C is also significant. If you compare two populations—one eating an apple a day and the other not—you should see a pattern of increased heart attack, stroke, and atherosclerosis in those not eating the apples, unless they had another dietary source for silicon and vitamin C. Yes, you would probably not need a doctor as often if your diet were adequate in these two nutrients, so richly present in the common apple.

MODERN MYTHS: MY FAVORITE SIX

A lot of ancient folklore has stood the test of time. Often, after a long period of scoffing, modern science has come to corroborate the folklore. In contrast, modern myths are often the products of science, directly or indirectly.

Modern Myth Number One: Putting Filters on Cigarettes Was Good for the Smoker

Wrong! Filter-tipped cigarettes have been around long enough for us to observe a declining death rate in those smokers who use them—if the rate is going to decline. But it hasn't happened. Filters do remove tars, keeping the carcinogens out of the lungs; but they allow the carbon monoxide to be absorbed even better! Some smokers use filters "for their health"—but smoke more and inhale deeper to meet the needs of their addiction. More carbon monoxide is absorbed by the smoker—increasing deaths due to heart attack. So filters did reduce the number of lung tumors; but this is more than offset by the increased deaths due to atherosclerosis.

Modern Myth Number Two: Margarine Is Better for You Than Butter

Wrong! Animal studies show that margarine is *more* atherogenic than butter if the margarine contains *trans*-fat formed during the partial hydrogenation of vegetable oils. Except for imported brands, it does!

Modern Myth Number Three: Worry about a High Cholesterol Level in Your Blood

Wrong! Worry more about a *low* level of the protective HDL-cholesterol in your blood. Kannel and Castelli have recently modified their conclusions from the Framingham study to include the more important measurement of HDL-cholesterol.[5] The *higher* the HDL-cholesterol the *better!* It goes up with your levels of physical activity, beer drinking, and vitamin C. HDL goes *down* with smoking and obesity, of course. Also, you should note that raising the HDL-cholesterol also raises the total cholesterol, because the total includes HDL and other types of cholesterol. Therefore, eating whole eggs can be good for you if it raises your total cholesterol by increasing the *HDL* fraction. (And it does.)

The hazard of watching your total cholesterol is this: You do things to lower your HDL (like stop drinking beer and start smoking), and watch your total cholesterol go down and think you have helped. If your total goes down because your HDL goes down, you are in more trouble. If the total cholesterol goes up because the HDL is going up, you are in less trouble.[6]

George Mann of Vanderbilt University has published extensive essays on the foolishness of trying to change your total blood cholesterol by watching only the cholesterol in your diet.[7]

However, modern "myths" die hard; and you will continue

to see semisynthetic substitutes for wholesome natural foods like eggs and whole milk. The oil and spread industries have much to gain by keeping the cholesterol "myth" alive; and we have much to lose!

Modern Myth Number Four: Beer Is Bad for You

Wrong! Beer has silicon, so it lowers the incidence of silicon-deficiency diseases such as heart attack and arthritis. Beer raises protective HDL-cholesterol, protecting against heart attack. Beer is the best way to prevent kidney stones and runner's hematuria.

Kidney stones form when the urine in the kidney becomes too concentrated because of dehydration. Dehydration, even during exercise with sweating, causes temporary kidney shutdown. Salts in the kidney dry out and form stones when the kidney stops flushing urine through. It takes two or three times as much fluid to keep the kidneys working during exercise as at rest. Beer works specifically by blocking the anti-diuretic hormone (ADH) from the brain, thus keeping the kidneys working; so it takes much less beer than any other liquid to get the same urine output. Therefore, as you run, your kidneys continue to flush urine through, keeping salts in solution and preventing stone formation.

Also, with a little urine in your bladder during the run, the bladder has a cushion to protect it from bruising—bruised bladder is caused by bouncing an empty bladder around while running. The bruises bleed—giving the runner red urine—called *runner's hematuria*. Beer prevents that by keeping a little urine in the bladder all the time.

Modern Myth Number Five: Eggs Are Bad for You

Nonsense. Egg protein is so perfect that all other proteins are measured against it. Egg protein is about 95 percent available for human use. The protein in other foods is less efficient, and you need more of it to match the amount in an egg, calorie for calorie. The cholesterol in an egg is not dangerous when it comes with the protein in the egg white. There are *no* human or animal studies showing hazards in *whole egg!*

Modern Myth Number Six: Peanuts Have Too Much Fat

Nonsense! *Whole* seeds and nuts, like whole grain, supply a wide variety of nutrients along with the natural oils. Of course there are studies with *extracted oils* that show diseases can be produced; but *extracted* calories of any kind have been used to cause a wide variety of diseases. If any refined calorie is present at 40 percent of the diet, it displaces a number of vital nutrients—and the deficiencies caused by the lack of these nutrients can look like a disease. However, no one has produced disease using *whole* seeds or nuts.

MARATHONING FOLKLORE

Then there's the body of folklore growing up about long-distance runners. True or false?

Folklore: Marathoners Burn Fat More Easily

True. Under the microscope, "friendly fat" containing high levels of the EFA linoleic acid has a different appearance from the unfriendly fats in burned grease and hydrogenated *trans*-fat.[8] This can be used to support the view that marathon runners have an almost magic ability to eat the right fatty fuel for the race. It is very healthy to have high linoleic-acid levels in your body tissues, and marathoners' high levels probably explain why they do not suffer from heart attack, stroke, and the other diseases of old age.

Folklore: Marathoners Need Extra Vitamin C

True. Autopsy sections of both arteries and tendons show low-ascorbic-acid injury before symptoms appear. Injuries, such as a torn Achilles tendon or degenerating knee cartilage, can be predicted in those who do heavy training mileage without *pounds* of fresh raw fruit and vegetables every day, or supplemental vitamin C.

Folklore: Marathoners Need Extra Vitamin E

Probably. Animal studies show that the need for vitamin E increases with the increased intake of polyunsaturated fats. Also, the need for E increases as the level of polyunsaturated fat increases in the tissue. In some individuals, the level of linoleic acid may be as low as 2 percent of body fat, while this polyunsaturated fatty acid may be as high as 50 percent of body fat in others.[9] Therefore, marathoners who use fat for fuel and store more linoleic acid will need more vitamin E.

In autopsy, low vitamin E shows up as the "sticky platelet" lesions in the heart muscle, associated with sudden death. Adequate vitamin E should keep platelets from becoming too sticky. I have seen two runners die with sticky platelets; as you recall, one smoked (a source of oxides to destroy E) and the other ate two charbroiled steaks a day (another source of oxides). Since vitamin E protects the polyunsaturated fatty fuel of the marathoner, I assume he has adequate vitamin E as long as he is capable of running the distance.

Folklore: Marathoners Need Extra Silicon

True. Autopsy evidence of low-silicon injury consists of a fragmentation of the tissue in the arterial wall. Similar changes occur in the injured tendons. How can you know if you're eating enough silicon-rich food? Simple. If your stools float, there is enough silicon in your diet.

There is good autopsy evidence to support the folklore of running: the increased needs for EFAs, vitamin C, vitamin E, and silicon. In a field as controversial as nutrition, the sportsman is wise in following his individual cravings. Food is important; and only whole foods can really be trusted.

TEN

Eat Your Way to the Finish Line

Runners have an expression for a competitor who "conks out" toward the end of a race: he "dies." The event is no longer exhilarating; it's hell for him. Something similar happens to the old person—or one not so old!—who is forced to spend his declining years in a hospital bed or nursing home. That's no way to come to the finish of a race. Ideally, the Whole Life Diet will carry you through life with an exhilarating feeling up to the very finish. What happens to you at the end of a race can give you a good clue to what awaits you when you're ninety.

It should be clear by now that the only solution to hospital rooms that cost $360 a day is to avoid them—at all costs. If the health industry isn't moving toward preventive medicine it's on a collision course. And by preventive medicine I mean a "health watch," as explained in Chapter Four: not just early diagnosis of disease, but dietary prevention of disease. In this chapter I'd like to look at diet from the aspect of the stress of competition. Preventing injury in a race tells us something about preventing disease in the stress of life.

If I am looking through my microscope at an artery I can tell a lot about the diet of the individual. If the "pavement" *endothelial* cells are missing from the inside of the artery: low vitamin C. If there are sticky platelets everywhere: low vitamin E. If the fat is inflamed and unfriendly: low EFAs. If the tissue is falling apart because of weak ground substance or collagen: low silicon and/or low vitamin C. All of these factors must be adequate in order for the individual to *be able* to cover the twenty-six-mile marathon distance on foot. Therefore, this minimum threshold distance is a good index of your diet. If you can't walk twenty-six miles, then you should examine your diet very closely. The proper diet keeps your body young and enables you to cover the distance. A poor diet *ages* your body and prevents you from being a marathon finisher!

I will be repeating many of the basic facts about the Whole Life Diet here—but from a different perspective. The competitive person automatically and willingly puts stress on his shoulders. That's another matter. Competition is his motivation. The aerobics generation has taught us that we can be equally motivated for our *well-being*. I am more interested in surviving the race than in winning. Death during the race certainly ruins the day for everyone!

To keep this chapter in perspective, we should remember the things that can injure or kill the athlete. Diet is important in each of the following conditions.

Silent Heart Disease—A hazard for many. But runners with significant narrowing of their coronary arteries are running marathons. I have run with over a hundred such cardiac athletes. If they have a cardiologist for a coach, they will run a safe race by keeping an eye on their pacing. And diet dictates pacing.

Heat Illness—Exertion-induced heat illness can affect many organs: brain, kidneys, liver, and heart. Usually the runners who are untrained and trying too hard are the ones who need medical treatment at the end of a race on hot days. Correct pacing and fluid intake prevent this.

Smoking—Tobacco use can cause irregular heartbeats—arrhythmia—when combined with vigorous exercise. Stop smoking first!

Carbon Monoxide—"Secondhand" smoke ties up your hemo-globin and reduces your oxygen-carrying capacity, reducing your work capacity. Keep out of rooms with smokers!

THE FIRST DIETARY RULE FOR RUNNERS: RESTORE THE POTASSIUM/SODIUM BALANCE

Low potassium, or *hypokalemia,* has caused more than one long-distance runner's heart to stop. Usually, the condition is easily treated if the runner is resuscitated and brought to the hospital in time. All that is needed is fluid replacement including the needed potassium.

Why do runners get low potassium?

The normal range of potassium in the blood is from 3.5 to 5.5 mEq/L (the standard measurement). The kidneys manage to keep it in the normal range *if* the diet contains enough fluids and potassium-rich foods. When you go on a long training run, your muscles get warmed up and lose some of their potassium temporarily. It leaks out into your blood, but returns to the inside of the muscle cell when you are resting. So, it would not be unusual for a marathoner to have a blood potassium above 5.5 during a fifteen-mile run, and below 3.5 twelve hours later when he was resting.

Kidneys will dump potassium when the blood level is above 5.5, and sweat carries some potassium from the body. So there is a daily need for new potassium. This is easily met when a *raw* diet is eaten, because most foods are naturally rich in potassium. However, milling, cooking, and food processing remove potassium and add sodium.

It is the *ratio* of potassium to sodium that causes most of the problems, because our bodies are designed to eat a raw diet, saving the sodium, which is scarce in nature, and dumping the potassium, which is too plentiful in natural foods.

However, modern foods are processed or cooked so that the ratio is reversed, abnormally high in sodium and low in potassium—dangerous! Dr. Hugh Trowell of England has studied the Kikuyu of Kenya and observed that they had no hypertension in 1930 *because* of their hunter-gatherer diet—high in potassium and low in sodium. Modern Kenyans add salt (containing sodium) to their foods and suffer from hypertension.[1]

Examples of this reversal of the sodium/potassium (Na/K) ratio are easy to find, because almost any type of cooking will remove potassium, and table salt (NaCl) is a common source of extra sodium. During boiling, cabbage potassium drops from 390 to 160 milligrams per deciliter.

Bread has a Na/K ratio of 540/100, or five to one; but in whole-meal flour it is 3/360, or roughly one to a hundred! Our ancestor, the hunter-gatherer before bread entered his diet, ate grain with a hundred times more potassium than sodium. His kidnys had to dump potassium and save sodium. Evolution hasn't allowed us time enough to adjust to dumping sodium and saving potassium, so we get into trouble. We either have too much sodium and high blood pressure, or we exercise to get into shape and lose too much potassium and get hypokalemia.

Other foods show a similar shift in the Na/K ratio in processing.

Uncooked *peas* have a Na/K ratio of 1/340, but canning peas changes it to 230/130. The magnitude of the ratio change is about the same as that seen in the grain-to-bread change—six hundredfold!

Beef, uncooked, has Na/K of 55/280, but corned beef has Na/K of 950/140. The ratio changes from 1/5 to 9/1.

Dietary precautions for runners would include eating as many raw items as possible. Whole cereals, all fruits, and most vegetables have ten to a hundred times more potassium than sodium. Beer also has more potassium than sodium. Taking two or three days a week off from running will allow the body a chance to replace lost potassium. Also, ritual eating of certain foods will set a safety pattern: for instance, one banana or tomato every six miles.

Most runners never realize why they crave certain foods or gravitate to three-days-on, two-days-off training a week. It's the potassium!

THE SECOND DIETARY RULE FOR RUNNERS: PICTURE WHAT FATS AND SMOKE DO TO YOUR BLOOD!

Cardiac patients who already have narrowed vessels and old scars in the heart will have to be more careful than other runners, since they can get into trouble more easily. Some medications, like diuretics and certain drugs for hypertension, may make them more prone to lose potassium, and they should be even more careful with their diet.

A meal high in any fat will cause a temporary rise of fats in the blood, as they are moved from the gut to the liver, The blood will look creamy for a few hours after a high-fat meal, so we can expect the excess fat to cause some trouble with the blood's oxygen-carrying capacity. Some cardiac patients can actually get chest pain *at rest* when they eat a fatty meal. Others get into trouble only when they exercise, because their blood carries less oxygen while the fat level is high. Fortunately, most of the cardiac arthletes I have run with have been educated by their cardiologist-coaches and nurses. They know more about their hearts than you could find in most books.

Smoking will tie up some of the *hemoglobin*—the part of blood that carries the oxygen—with carbon monoxide, leaving it less free to carry oxygen. This reduces the amount of exercise you can handle, of course. It also increases the hazards of eating a fatty meal, which further decreases oxygen-carrying capacity. No one should have a big cigar after a big steak dinner—especially someone with known heart disease.

Even if you share a closed room with a smoker you have to worry. Cardiac patients were exercised on a treadmill in a smoky room. With windows open they lost 20 percent of work capacity; with windows closed they lost 40 percent. Athletes will try to avoid the smoking sections of planes and trains for this reason. Even a beginner will instinctively avoid smoky places. This may be the result of his diet, since the EFA linoleic acid reacts with oxides in smoke, forming toxic lipid oxides, which are very irritating. Athletes who eat seeds, nuts, and grains have higher tissue levels of linoleic acid and therefore less tolerance for tobacco smoke.

That's right! The nonsmoker's annoyance with smoke isn't just some sort of elitist reaction. The more you train, the more intolerable smoke becomes. This fact explains why joggers always seem to give up smoking. *It's perhaps the best way to stop!*

THE THIRD DIETARY RULE FOR RUNNERS: EDUCATE YOUR STOMACH AND LISTEN TO IT

If you crave something, eat it! It probably contains something you need. If the need is filled, the cravings should cease. Unfortunately, sedentary people have very dumb stomachs. It's not their fault; society can be blamed. By removing the necessary exercise from our lives, we are left with yesterday's calories *unburned*. While our bodies try to store these unburned calories, our stomachs are empty—so we eat without purpose. If we had burned those calories, we would have created an empty gas tank to guide our taste buds. If we had used anaerobic exercise and burned carbohydrates, we would crave carbohydrates. If we had used aerobic exercise, beyond the first hour, we would have burned some carbohydrate and some fat—creating a craving for a mixed diet. If the heat of the exercise had caused loss of salts in sweat, we would find that salty things tasted unusually good. The minerals and other micronutrients also trigger their own particular cravings.

Exercise is the key to raising the IQ of your stomach and taste buds. Marathon running, because it is associated with protection from the aging process, creates the smartest taste buds I have seen. Many of the items craved by these long-distance runners have been used in animal studies to protect against atherosclerosis and other diseases of old age.

However, society has tricked us in many ways. Foods we crave may not have the needed nutrient that triggered the cravings because the nutrients have been *processed out* of it! That is why marathon runners crave *whole* fruit and vegetables, cheap local beer, nuts, onions, garlic, whole grains. They are allowing their stomachs and their taste buds to select their menu.

We're at a point where we can consider the import of some of the nutritional truisms of our day. In an article in the *New York Times,* Dr. Clayton Thomas, a consultant to the aerospace people, an internist, and officially the vice-president of medical affairs for Tampax, Inc., was quoted as saying, "While fresh foods may offer an esthetic advantage to some people, in general they are no better nutritionally than processed. Overcooking and improper storage . . . can give them a distinct disadvantage as far as nutritional content is concerned." [2] I hope the discussion of potassium and fats and unburned carbohydrates in this chapter dispels that sort of cynical appraisal. That's enough, but I've mentioned plenty of other reasons why fresh foods are essential. Until now, no one has considered the impact of the aerobics movement on diet.

AEROBIC ATHLETES *ARE* DIFFERENT METABOLICALLY

Marathon runners burn body fat more easily than untrained individuals do.[3] These metabolic studies were done *at rest,* indicating that marathon runners can just sit there and be smug, knowing that they are burning more body fat than the rest of the sedentary population!

Don Kalmar has shown that marathon runners actually burn fat more easily than they burn glycogen. What this means is the metabolic pathways for obtaining energy from fat are more highly developed in athletes who use fat for fuel during their sport. Kalmar took trained runners: marathoners (aerobic) and middle-distance runners (anaerobic). He measured their maximum oxygen uptakes in the usual way first—when the runners were well rested. During this test, they could use muscle glycogen for fuel. By measuring the respiratory quotient (RQ), he confirmed that they were burning glycogen. The respiratory quotient is the ratio between oxygen consumed and carbon dioxide given off during exercise:

$$RQ = \frac{Vol.\ CO_2}{Vol.\ O_2}$$

The RQ for carbohydrates (glycogen) is 1.0. Kalmar's runners showed very high maximum oxygen uptakes, indicating that all were very well trained. He recorded each runner's oxygen uptake at the RQ of 1.0 (on glycogen).

Then he removed all glycogen from the muscles with a fourteen-hour fast and a fourteen-mile run. (Some of the middle-distance men had to walk part of the depletion run; however, it used 1,400 calories of energy, enough to remove all muscle glycogen.)

Now all runners were burning fat. The RQ for fat is 0.7. This means that for every volume of oxygen taken in, only 0.7 volumes of carbon dioxide are given off. When he repeated the maximum oxygen uptakes on fat fuel, the marathoners showed an *increase* over their previous readings, while the middle-distance runners had a *decrease* in the amount of work they could do. The oxygen uptakes are measured on a treadmill—i.e., the oxygen uptake for the work of running is measured when you are running at your maximum rate. Marathoners, who race twenty-six-mile distances, can do more work on fat than on glycogen. They can actually speed up their pace at the eighteen-mile mark, because fat is a more efficient fuel for them. Middle-distance runners race at six miles and less, using glycogen, and they slow down when they switch to fatty fuel.

Both Kalmar's work during exercise and the report on marathoners at rest show that they *are* metabolically different. They have a more efficient pathway to burn fat than sedentary individuals. Also, Kalmar shows that not all types of exercise can enlarge your fat-burning pathway. In fact, anaerobic ice-hockey players had a less favorable pattern of blood lipids than the aerobic long-distance runners.[4] I expect all metabolic studies to show a difference between aerobic and anaerobic sportsmen because of their different sources of energy during their sport activities.

THE LONG RUN

The twenty-four-hour run is something anyone can do. You just enter and go as far as you want in twenty-four hours. One sociable fellow signed up the first year in Hawaii to get the fancy shirt, and he ran one mile! Perhaps that *was* the longest run in his life; who knows?

If you contemplate a great physical effort, your first concern is nutrition that will help *performance*. I encourage my teenage children and my friends to enter ultra-long running events like the twenty-four-hour run and the fifty-mile run simply because they are so long that they are slow and sociable. If you can stay awake for twenty-four hours and walk a steady two miles an hour, you'll exceed forty miles and perhaps reach fifty! Experienced ultramarathoners can give you advice about training, shoes, and pacing; but I will outline the nutritional concepts I found useful.

First, plan your effort so that you arrive at the twenty-hour mark fresh, rested, with plenty of water and carbohydrate in your body. If you are exhausted at twenty hours, those who are fresh can continue for four more hours and greatly exceed your eventual distance. Plan to walk nine hours, sleep one, walk nine more, nap again for an hour, then jog four. Eighteen hours of walking could total fifty-four miles, plus four hours of jogging, another twenty miles or so—total over seventy miles! And that allows for two hours of napping.

Anyone who has ever run ultradistance events, and survived to run the next day, will tell you that he had a secret of some kind—fluids, diet, pills, yoga—that made the difference between success and failure.

The first thing you must avoid, of course, is *death*. Death can come in many forms when you exceed your previous maximum distance, but most start with dehydration and kidney shutdown. Fluid intake must be paced with your sweat and urine losses. Drink enough to urinate often during the event. I aim for six rest stops in the one-day run—or once every four hours. If you have adequate urine output, it's almost impossible to get into trouble with heat or dehydration.

My favorite site for the twenty-four-hour run is on the island of Oahu, where the Primo Beer Company caters to the needs of over ten thousand runners once a year. The run is supported by the Honolulu YMCA Cardiac Rehabilitation Program, so the event is designed for slow joggers who are there to have a good time. It is very safe, with water stops and rest rooms only two miles apart. You run on a four-mile loop, so you can set up a camp where your handler can take proper care of you: timing laps, changing clothes, and fixing fluids and special foods.

What foods?

Eat what you crave! That is the first rule. I thought that I would crave salted peanuts after sweating and drinking beer for ten hours, but I didn't. My body was telling me not to think with my brain but rather to listen to my stomach and taste buds. My body needed certain key nutrients. They may have been peculiar to me; or many runners may have needed the same things. I observed myself and other runners. The nutrients I detected included: silicon, carnitine, thiamin, ascorbic acid, and other *water*-soluble vitamins. No one craved EFAs!

And everyone seemed to crave living things. Some of them were sprouts, acidophilus, and yeast. They're easy to provide. It takes three or four days to fill your *sprouter* with crisp little plants rich in all the water-soluble vitamins. All runners ate sprouts. *Acidophilus* cultures appeared as kefir and yogurt. This helps keep the gut flora friendly. Yeast arrived as brewer's-yeast tablets and sourdough bread. Feed your *sourdough starter* the night before, and bake a couple of loaves of sourdough bread just before the event.

Chicken soup is rich in *carnitine*. Keep a pot of soup on the camp stove during the cool night hours of the race. Add crisp chopped vegetables just before you are ready to eat some. The carnitine is a B vitamin that helps you to burn fatty acids.

Silicon is present in the beer. You can keep a pot of hot alfalfa tea brewing at night; drink it with honey when you're cold.

Extra *calories* in the form of brown rice seemed popular

after about eighteen hours. I put my rice in my soup. Bread and beer are also rich sources of calories, mostly carbohydrate.

Take a gram of sodium *ascorbate* (vitamin C) every six miles. Few runners ate significant amounts of fruit during the event, but all craved large amounts the day *after* the run.

Fluid intake should be adequate to stimulate urination—about a quart an hour. In my case, half of the fluid was water, about a fourth was soup or tea, and a fourth was beer or soft drinks.

Total *calories* should match the energy cost of the event—about 5,000 calories for those doing fifty miles.

If you plan your strategy correctly, you should be able to cover a greater distance every year. If someone asks you what your secret is, just say: I only eat living things during the run!

The sourdough starter was alive until you cooked the bread; the chicken and vegetables were alive until you cooked the soup!

Stay away from *pills* and other synthetic items. The pill may not dissolve when you need it, or too many pills may suddenly give you more of something than you want. Potassium pills taken during a marathon will pass right through if you get diarrhea. On the other hand, they might dissolve in your gut and raise your blood potassium too high and kill you. Remember, blood potassium goes up during exercise! Caffeine is also available in pills. I have seen one runner require medical treatment because he took three caffeine tablets during a marathon. He was lucky—he could have died.

Running is natural; and a raw diet is natural. If you are going to tamper with these rules you should know what you are doing. *It's dangerous to remain sedentary; and it's dangerous to process your food.* You should get a doctor's evaluation if you want to remain sedentary; and you should *think* before you process all nutrients out of your diet.

If you plan your strategy correctly—for racing *and* for living—you should be able to cover a greater distance every year. For many years.

ELEVEN

How to Buy Health in the Supermarket – Or Grow Your Own!

You will have guessed by now that I have little trust in the supermarket. You're right: I think the supermarket can kill you. But I think it also can cure you. The difference is that it's not out to cure you; it's out to kill you. You're its enemy.

These are strong words. But I don't mean to imply that your store manager, or your checkout person, or your produce manager is after you. It's the very structure of the store, the selling process, the corporate economics of the supermarket chain, and ultimately the economics of the suppliers that make you an enemy instead of a friend. Safeway used to advertise, "Since we're neighbors, let's be friends!" Safeway is right—they are as much a friend as they are a neighbor.

I mean no insult to any particular store. A&P, Grand Union, Lucky, Gristede's, Mayfair, and even your local mom-and-pop operation are no different. They all stock what's selling. And what's selling is unfortunately controlled more by national advertising and market economics than by buyer preference. I don't agree with economists like John Kenneth Galbraith that national advertisers have their way with consumers if they spend enough in the "right" ways; it's not always true. But the fact is that *the profit motive* does indeed dictate a whole class of goods that are promotable but only apparently good for you.

Most of us, I'm afraid, are optimists when it comes to economics. We tend to believe that the many changes in food processing and packaging result in a better food product on our tables. Fast, efficient, innocuous food—that's our goal. After all, there are more important things in life than eating. We're a busy people. "What's wrong with sugar?" William Rusher asks in his nationally syndicated column on sugarcoated breakfast cereals. "Any breakfast is better than no breakfast." If the trends are to frozen dinners and staleproof breads, so much the better for the quality of our lives in other areas.

In this short chapter I don't pretend to be able to change this way of thinking—if that's the way you think. But I'd like at least to offer food for your thought. In our recent history there was indeed a turning point in what you and I could buy to feed ourselves. Consider what the chairman of the Council on Children, Media, and Merchandising, Robert Choate, said before Congress in 1972:

> The military requirements of World War II produced a host of food technology innovations. Meals for our armed forces had to stand storage for months. Snacks called K and C rations became substitute meals. Drinks from powdered ingredients and eggs and milk in a dry-pack cardboard box came to be common. . . . Processed foods, using basically inexpensive materials that were coaxed into supposedly fascinating new shapes, colors, and smells came to be advertised and glorified out of proportion to their nutritional contribution.[1]

What I'm saying is that we were induced to buy a whole new *class* of food, not just one brand over another. And this class of food was dictated, not by greedy industrialists or heartless brand-managers, but by a technology that answered the needs of postwar economics. If cars could be mass-produced, why not food?

Nutritionist Jean Mayer spelled out the result in chilling detail: Because of pressure on food suppliers to become an "agribusiness," manufacturers naturally turned food into a *product*. The inevitable, Mayer says, is that "they are going to look for cheaper and cheaper sources of raw materials. The cheapest sources of raw materials are sugar and hydrogenated vegetable fat." [2] And that's why we are forced to eat them. That's why the manufactured food product isn't just a convenience, or a way of making more food generally available. No—the manufactured food product is merely a business transaction. It's really not a food at all.

In any discussion of this sort you will read that "consumer demands" have led to strawberries in the winter (frozen packages) and that "consumer choices" have led to canned ravioli and tacos. Modern food technology has made all of this possible. As in any debate, a kernel of truth can be claimed by either side of any proposition about consumer preferences and food merchandising. It's true: we have hundreds of good foods available now through freezing and canning that we didn't have prior to World War II. But let's examine both sides of this story:

1. Food processing of any kind is damaging to food values, often to an extent that makes the processing self-defeating. That is, we receive the illusion of a good food without the food! I've mentioned many examples. Yet the offical USDA position is that canned vegetables, for example, are nutritionally equivalent to fresh!

2. Preservatives in processed foods are necessary—for health and for economics! As we will see, I don't find nitrites and things like BHT and BHA to be the real villains.

3. You *can* influence what's on the shelves by your buying habits. But remain a skeptic. Example: granola was ridiculed by the large manufacturers when it was still a "health-nut" food. But when it became a big seller, they all went into production (with their own doctored product, to be sure).

4. You don't have to be a "health nut" and ignore the supermarket to find good food values. But you must be strong.

In this chapter I'm going to explore the *practical* options you have. As we've seen throughout the book, foods can be considered to be good, bad, or indifferent. Hydrogenated fats and noncalorie sweeteners are dangerous *in themselves*. Empty-calorie foods such as white bread, sugar, and alcohol are indifferent: they become dangerous only if you don't replace the nutrients they rob you of. The best foods contain my *basic three nutrients*: vitamin C, silicon, essential fatty acids. Keep an eye on these and all the other nutrients will follow. Any food that has an essential fatty acid, for example, must also contain amino acids—proteins—because processing would remove the more fragile fatty acids first.

WHOLE FOODS: YOUR GOAL

Walk through several supermarkets with a checklist. How many staples can be bought whole?

Cereal grains: I think that a flour mill should have been the key kitchen appliance, not the refrigerator. Whole grains keep very well in their hulls, and can be ground to flour as needed.

The best *bread* is from your own kitchen, where you have control over ingredients. The safest place in the supermarket to buy bread is the refrigerated section—if it's there, it's probably less refined and has fewer artificial substances added. Read the label. Avoid anything with hydrogenated shortenings.

Breakfast cereals: Aren't all bad. There's nothing wrong with oats. When Quaker Oats first rolled them for cooking, the effect was a rise in the popularity of breakfast hot cereal. Shredded wheat, designed to be eaten hot or cold, also appeared in the late nineteenth century. Both contained some of the natural antioxidant, vitamin E, in the wheat-germ oils. Puffed wheat came along in the early 1900s. Kellogg brought wheat flakes, and Post added Grape Nuts, a combination of wheat and barley.

The decline in the incidence of stomach cancer can be explained by the rise in popularity of these breakfast cereals in America. About 1947, another source of dietary antioxidants appeared—BHT, a food preservative discussed in the next section. This was associated with a further decline in gastric cancer rates.

So the whole-grain breakfast cereals are essentially beneficial. But other breakfast cereals are hard to justify when you read the labels. The added synthetic vitamins may act just like the natural vitamins, but I worry about all the other nutrients that were originally removed when the grain was processed: bran with minerals, EFAs, protein, etc. I just do not trust the chemists who designed the boxed foods. They may have left something out that I need. They're only chemists.

Some of the boxed cereals taste very good, but it seems odd to sprinkle wheat germ and bran on an expensive "cereal" from a box. It's more logical to buy whole grain groats and make hot cereal at home.

Other boxed cereals have so much sugar that I consider them to be a form of candy—expensive, but with no food value. The three key nutrients I watch are absent!

Dairy products: Whole milk, eggs, yogurts, and cheeses can be found in all cities. But read the labels—some yogurts will pass for candy. Skim milk has the fat removed, but I am not afraid of milk fat, since *whole* milk lowers blood cholesterol. When fat is skimmed off, the natural vitamin D is removed. One of the reasons I drink milk is to get vitamin D, and I don't trust synthetic vitamin D completely.

Meat: Chicken and fish have good protein and less saturated fat than the red meats. The red meats should be used to flavor soups and starchy dishes, not for a whole meal in themselves. Most of the calories in marbled beef come from fat, not protein!

Vegetables: Fresh is best, but when winter comes you may have to go to frozen or canned. Nutrients are lost in every step of processing. Watch prices, because fresh produce will usually be cheaper *per serving*. The root vegetables (potatoes, onions, beets, etc.) can be bought in bulk and stored well in a root drawer at home. The leafy vegetables wilt quickly and their prices fluctuate with the seasons.

Fruit: Here, again, fresh is best. As with leafy vegetables, you are after vitamin C and other water-soluble vitamins. These nutrients are quickly lost in processing. Juices made from concentrate may have *no* biologically available vitamin C! Also, the fruit pectin, a source of silicon, is removed from most juices. If you enjoy fruit juice, it is best to buy a juicing machine; get one that leaves most of the pulp in the juice. Dried fruit can be eaten at any time of year, and it contains pectin, but little vitamin C.

Seeds and nuts: The natural sources of EFAs and vitamin E are seeds—living things designed by nature to sleep through the winter and then spring to life. They contain essential fatty acids. Along with whole grains and eggs, the seeds and nuts should be eaten regularly. However, the roasted nuts are killed and have lost their EFAs. Raw, whole nuts can be obtained in their shells at bulk prices. They keep well, and make safe snacks.

CALORIE GOALS IN A DIET

The bulk of your caloric intake should come from plants (whole grain cereals and root vegetables like potatoes). If you get them whole and prepare them in your own kitchen, they can provide all the EFAs, vitamins C and E, and silicon you need; and the price is right! Expensive fruits, nuts, dairy products, and meats can be added for variety, offering a luxury of colors, flavors, and extra nutrients.

As we have seen in the case of the Pritikin low-fat diet, excess calories are no problem if you eat whole foods. The easiest way to count calories is to ignore the numbers and concentrate on the right foods.

FOOD ADDITIVES: WHO'S RIGHT?

When anything is added to food, it is an additive. Some are necessary and safe. Others are dangerous but serve a useful purpose. Still others are dangerous and their use is merely cosmetic.

Food coloring has no essential function in nutrition. Many of the cheap synthetic dyes that have been used in foods are now banned because they cause cancer in lab animals. Other dyes are still being used, but they are suspect. I would avoid anything with a red *dye* added.

A number of natural pigments are being used. If they are manufactured from food sources, then I don't worry so much.

Beets, for example, are a source of *anthocyans,* the pigment that gives them their red color. All green leaves contain *xanthophyll* and *carotene,* so they should be safe coloring agents.

Nitrites can form *nitrosamines,* cancer-causing agents. However, nitrites are used in curing meat to prevent the growth of deadly *Clostridium botulinum,* a cause of food poisoning that can be quickly fatal. *Botulism* was a big threat in the old days when home canning was common. It sparked the growth of the canning industry, because the critical temperature needed to kill the germs and sterilize the food was difficult in homes before the pressure cooker was developed.

I am divided on the use of nitrites. Natural substitutes related to vitamin C (*ascorbate* and *erythorbate*) are now being used, but our own gut produces more nitrites than we were getting in cured meat. (By taking several grams of sodium ascorbate—a soluble form of ascorbic acid—each day we can block the formation of these nitrosamines in our gut.) Nitrites are dangerous, certainly, but botulism is even more dangerous; the organism is everywhere and it grows readily at the temperatures at which cured meat is stored.

Antioxidants. Vitamins C and E, the natural antioxidants, are beneficial; even artificial antioxidants are probably safe, and may actually be very good for us. BHT and BHA are commonly added to any food where spoilage by oxidation is a problem (whole wheat and unpolished rice products). BHT stands for *butylated hydroxytoluene;* BHA is *butylated hydroxyanisol.* They act like vitamin E, preventing oxidation of EFAs. BHT was used in animals as an anti-aging agent; and in work done by Dr. Harman of the University of Nebraska, it did prolong the mean life span of mice.[3]

Toxic free radicals (formed from EFAs during vitamin E deficiency) have been implicated in the aging process; and BHT is one of the antioxidants that prevents the formation of free radicals. So I am not afraid of BHT and BHA.

Ascorbic acid is being used to prevent enzymatic browning of fruits and potatoes. This is sort of like using lemon juice for the same purposes at home: safe.

Mold inhibitors, such as propionate and sorbate, are quite harmless and very necessary. An ounce of Swiss cheese contains enough natural propionate to protect two pounds of bread from mold. Mold inhibitors are a very cheap way to keep bread safe— a penny's worth will protect about a hundred loaves. They should also be used with peanuts, rice, corn, and soybeans, which can support a mold that produces highly toxic carcinogens. In this area, I think *more* food additives should be used!

Sugar, sucrose, is the leading food additive in America. We each consume about our full body weight in sugar each year! Sugar is a food, and it does prevent spoilage of jams, jellies, and other things. (Most bacteria and fungi will not grow in sugar!) However, it is certainly an empty calorie—devoid of EFAs, silicon, and vitamins. It has been called pure energy by the candy industry; but we have learned that calories are not available for energy unless they are covered by nutrients (vitamins, amino acids, etc.). The sugar calorie does not satisfy hunger for nutrients, and is probably the biggest contributor to obesity. If you are overweight, you can avoid all sources of sucrose without the loss of a single nutrient.

Salt is a common additive also. However, salt is sodium chloride (NaCl)—and the average sodium intake is too high relative to the potassium intake, as discussed elsewhere. Therefore, table salt is dangerous; it burdens the kidneys and causes fatal high blood pressure in some people.

Read labels and avoid taking too much salt. Some "potato chips" are not sliced potato at all, just potato starch plus grease, salt, and artificial flavorings and colorings—a synthetic snack that tastes good but adds no nutrients to the diet! Many snack foods use the *name* of a perfectly good food source, like "corn" or "potato," but offer nothing but a synthetic treat with too much sodium.

Monosodium glutamate (MSG) is a salt of one of the commonest amino acids, glutamic acid. Wheat protein is about 30 percent glutamate. This salt is used to bring out the flavor of foods. Like all sources of sodium, it should be watched. Hypertensive patients should limit sodium intake. However, as an additive it is no more dangerous than table salt.

GROW YOUR OWN LIVING THINGS

Although some additives are all right, even beneficial, it's best to stick to the basic rule as much as possible: Eat only living things. Since it's sometimes hard to buy them, you should consider growing your own.

Bread is central, and if you make it yourself from whole ingredients, it's good. It has living yeast in it, and is, in a sense, alive until it hits the oven. Baking bread at home involves grinding grain, getting flour all over your hands with the kneading, and baking. The yeast is alive, and must be treated gently— no harsh chemicals or sudden temperature changes. I'd advise you to watch someone else bake bread before trying it yourself. It takes experience to recognize the correct texture during kneading so you don't add too much or too little flour.

Before trying bread, you may find it easier to attempt simpler projects like sprouting and yogurt-making. Both involve growing a living thing into food. And if you keep a yeast starter (to raise the bread), bees (for honey), and a goat (for milk), you'll have most of the ingredients to go with the flour you grind yourself. Of course you don't have to raise all of it yourself, but each thing you do grow will improve the final product.

Sprouts for Fresh Vitamins

Sprouting is made simple by following the printed instructions in each small package of "sprouting" seeds. Your job is to wash them, soak them in water overnight, and spread them evenly in the clean sprouting chamber. A wide-mouth jar will do—put a cheesecloth over the mouth with a rubber band for easy rinsing. Instructions call for rinsing about four times a day to remove the metabolites of the seeds. I use an upright sprouting chamber so the sprouts stand at attention and have bright-green tops. The chamber has mesh to hold the seeds over a removable bottom, which contains water. It's easy to rinse and change water. In about four days, alfalfa produces two-inch sprouts; they wake up a sandwich. Garbanzos (chick-peas), mung beans, and soybeans produce big sprouts that can be sautéed with onions and other vegetables. Rye and wheat can be sprouted and ground for bread recipes.

Sprouts can be used anywhere vegetables are used: in soups, egg casseroles, salads, and snacks. When they're hiking, backpackers can use rainwater to grow sprouts. If you're in a submarine or a space station, your sprouter can give you fresh vegetables every day, rich in water-soluble vitamins.

All right. You'll never be in a submarine; but ten years ago I never thought I'd see alfalfa sprouts in a supermarket, either. They're in the fresh-produce section—back against the walls.

Yogurt, with Friendly Bacteria

You could consider your *yogurt culture* a pet—bacterial in size. You buy this pet culture in your supermarket as a plain yogurt. Try several; all should contain living organisms. The flavors depend on the culture used; if you find one that you like use it for your starter.

A yogurt maker is a little incubator with room for several jars. It keeps the temperature just right for growing the yogurt culture—about 110° F—for three to five hours.

To make yogurt, scald all utensils to kill any wild bacteria—all you want growing is your pet. Bring a pot of milk to a boil. Watch it closely, and remove it as soon as the first foam appears. Mix a few spoonfuls of the pet-yogurt starter with the foam, and then wait for the milk to cool to lukewarm—if it is too hot, it will kill the starter. Mix in the starter and pour the mixture into the scalded jars. I use a yogurt maker, but a pan of 110-degree water will do. The jars have lids to keep wild germs out while the mixture thickens. After it's thick, put it in the refrigerator to slow down the bacteria.

Gelatin powder added to the warm milk makes the yogurt stiffer; so does powdered milk—both add protein. Yogurt is a handy way to add "life" to your dairy-food intake. It can be substituted for sour cream in many recipes. It's also a safe dessert—just add fruit.

The health benefits from live yogurt come from the B vitamins—both those made in the jar and those made in your intestine. The yogurt bacteria are very "friendly"; they continue to live in your gut and their metabolism produces useful nutrients for you.

Now Try Pet Yeast

Once you've made yogurt, you'll appreciate that the bacteria need special care for growth—sterile food and proper temperature. The same is true for yeasts. Beer is made from sprouted (malted) grain, yeast, and water. Bread is made of grain (which can be sprouted first if desired), yeast, and water. The nutrients produced by yeast growing on sprouted grain are very valuable—a very rich source of the water-soluble B-complex vitamins.

Pet yeast can be kept in a jar in your refrigerator. It needs to be fed once a week, and can provide an unlimited supply of yeast, called sourdough starter, for baking.

Capture your pet yeast at the supermarket: a package of dry yeast dissolved in a cup of lukewarm water. Wait 15 minutes and stir in one cup of whole-wheat flour. Pour into a scalded jar and let it feed for several days at room temperature. When it is growing well it will look bubbly. Keep it in the refrigerator until you need it for making bread.

Feed the pet yeast once a week with 2 cups of flour and 2 cups of water. Do not use metal utensils or the metal ions may kill it. Mix the starter and flour in a wooden or earthenware bowl. Let it sit overnight in a warm place to feed. The next morning you will have 3 cups of starter to use for bread, and one cup to return to the refrigerator. Feed again at the end of the week.

Honey or Sugar? Watch for Footprints!

An average beehive produces about a pound of honey each week. During extraction, the honey is removed by centrifugal force, and the wax comb is replaced inside the hive. The raw honey may contain bees, or parts of them. These can be removed with a cheesecloth filter without heating the honey. It takes time, but the honey is now clear enough for use. It has not been heated, so it is essentially what the bees use for their carbohydrate energy. I trust honey more than white sugar because of its importance in the beehive; I suspect it contains important micronutrients. When asked what honey has that table sugar doesn't have, I answer, "Bee footprints"!

Bee footprints may be more important than you think. How do we know that sugar has "safe levels" of insecticides or pollutants? Government agencies set standards and chemists check crops. It's all very technical. And science tries to protect us.

But when we use honey extracted and filtered at home, *nature* protects us. The bee is a delicate creature. She must survive to make the honey. If crops are sprayed with toxins, they flourish, but the bees die. Table sugar comes from plants that are very sturdy compared to the honey bee. Soil toxins are more likely to reach our table through sugar than honey.

Fewer calories of honey than of sugar are needed to flavor a loaf of bread. Many flavors lurk in the honey, depending upon the flowers from which the nectar was gathered.

Honey is expensive and in short supply—actually a luxury. That is what all sweeteners should be, luxuries, used only sparingly. We would all be more healthy if the supply of sweets were limited. Much of our nutritional trouble is caused by the tons of readily available, cheap, processed, white sugar. It has become a major source of calories—causing deficiencies in fiber, EFAs, and vitamins. If we had only honey for sweetening, we would all be better off; there just isn't enough to get us into trouble. Its strong flavor prevents us from eating too much.

Beekeeping is an interesting hobby, combining many skills. The modern beekeeper's suit is virtually stingproof. It is a biological treat to work the hives, fighting off ants and wax moths, building frames, catching the wild swarms, and watching over the brood. If the queen is lost you can even induce the workers to make a new one by feeding a young larva some royal jelly. Your hive is a good monitor of the local ecology; if someone sprays insecticide the bees die!

The Bassler Dream: The "Goat-Dog"

Owning a goat is as easy as having a large dog. The goat can give 10 percent of her body weight in milk each day. Her droppings look like tiny black marbles—and can be sold to neighbors for rose-garden fertilizer. She can be driven to the vet like a dog—in your car. She costs about the same as a dog, and her diet of grain and alfalfa is cheaper than dog food! All in all, she earns her keep with milk, gives one to three offspring a year for meat or sale as milkers, smells better than a dog, and won't bite the neighbors! All you have to do is milk her twice a day, give her a warm, dry bed (in the dog house), and learn to live with the alfalfa bales in your living room. Young goats are bottle-fed by their new owners to "imprint" them, so they grow up thinking the human is their mother—makes them very friendly!

Once you have your own goat, you don't have to wonder what is in your milk supply; just watch what the goat eats! Raw goat's milk is white—all of the yellow carotene is converted to colorless vitamin A by the goat. (Cow's milk has some vitamin A plus some carotene.) Goat's milk has smaller particles of fat, so very little cream rises to the top. In a sense, it has been homogenized inside the goat. People who are allergic to cow's milk can usually tolerate goat's milk, because the proteins, coming from a different species, are a bit different.

Bassler's "goat-dog" is, in fact, a living lesson in the production of food. And, I hope, a drastic way of pointing out how numbed we have become by our supermarket way of living. Nothing wrong with a dog—but have we forgotten why we had animals around in the first place?

Put Them All Together for Protein-Rich Bread

Once you've sprouted wheat, you will understand that the grain is a living thing containing all the nutrients required for life. The amino-acid content is a bit different from our human needs, but milk protein can fix that. Both milk and wheat protein come with a mixture of amino acids, rich in some and poor in others. Wheat is poor in two of the amino acids that milk is rich in. Thus, adding milk to wheat is a natural thing to do—increasing the amount of useful protein by almost 50 percent.

There are nine amino acids which humans cannot make; so we have to eat them. The protein machinery of our bodies needs all nine, and it can build new body protein only when all are present. Thus, when a food is deficient in one amino acid, the protein in that food cannot be used until the body finds the missing amino acid in another food item. By combining foods correctly, we can make a match of their weak and strong points, obtaining all of the needed amino acids efficiently, with a minimum of calories.

Along with the wheat and milk, yeast or sourdough starter will turn the wheat and milk into bread.

Sourdough Bread

(makes 2 loaves)

1 cup sourdough starter (feed your starter the night before)
2½ cups warm milk
2 tablespoons honey (up to 4 tablespoons optional)
1 tablespoon salt (less if you're limiting sodium intake)
6 cups whole-wheat flour (grind it the same day to preserve EFAs)

Beat all the ingredients except the flour. Use a large bowl. Mix in the flour by hand. Cover and let rise until size doubles— about 3 hours. Shape into 2 loaves. Knead them a little as you place them in oiled pans. Allow to rise about 1½ hours or until size doubles. Bake at 350° F for 30 minutes. Remove from pans to cool.

Never use shortening! Substitute whole milk for the *water plus fat* in the usual recipe.

Simple Bread

(makes 2 loaves)

2 tablespoons dry yeast
3 cups warm water
1 teaspoon honey—to feed the yeast
8 cups whole-wheat flour

Mix ½ cup water, honey, and yeast; leave it till frothy— about 10 minutes. Mix flour and water by hand, add yeast mixture, and shape into loaves as soon as kneading produces right texture. Allow to rise about double in size; then bake at 375° F for about 40 minutes.

Note: This bread is really a simple food—whole wheat.

Super Bread

"Super bread" should come with a balanced protein source (wheat plus milk), be high fiber (added bran), and have a very good flavor (honey plus raisins) without any hazardous refined calories or shortenings. It should be simple to make, keep well, and hold together for toasting and sandwich making.

The key to the flavor is the freshness of the flour. Grinding the wheat on baking day avoids rancid flour. Grinding with stones rather than steel avoids destructive heat. Motor-driven stone grinders for household use are available at about the same price range as a small stove or refrigerator. They should last a lifetime.

(makes 2 loaves)

6 cups wheat *grain;* grind into about 8 cups of flour
1 cup of raw miller's bran—"unprocessed"
½ cup raw honey
1 teaspoon salt
2 tablespoons dry yeast
¼ cup raisins—see "optional treats" below
3 cups warm milk—raw whole milk
½ cup warm water—to wake up yeast

Mix warm water, yeast, and a teaspoon of honey; let it foam. Mix warm milk and honey. Mix 3 cups flour and the salt into the milk-and-honey mixture by hand. Add the yeast mixture and bran. Mix. Knead. Gradually add flour until you have a stiff, sticky dough. Allow to rise in bowl under cloth until it doubles in size. Punch ·down on breadboard and flatten. Roll in the raisins and shape into loaves. Allow them to rise again, until double in size. Bake 30 minutes at 350° F.

Optional Treats: You can add other things with the raisins, such as apple slices, cinnamon-plus-sugar mixture, or other chopped dried fruits. The tops can be made crisp with a sprinkle of water in the oven; or glaze them by painting before baking with a mixture of a well-beaten egg and a teaspoon of water. The glaze is a good place to put designs of caraway or sesame seeds.

These optional treats can be used to give each loaf its own individuality. With lots of treats you have a nourishing "fruit and nut" loaf; with no treats you have a high-fiber, complete-protein bread for toast and sandwiches. Molasses, about a table-spoonful, can be added with the honey to increase the content of trace elements. Oatmeal or rye flour can be substituted for part of the whole-wheat flour for a slightly different texture and flavor.

YOUR "SUPERMARKET DUTY"

You'll understand my reluctance to give you absolute guide-lines for shopping in the supermarket. Tastes are so different—remember, you have your own bodyprint! You'll also understand the risk I'm taking in talking about making your own bread and growing your own sprouts. The risk is that I'll be considered some kind of a nut! Adelle Davis took that risk and wasn't vin-dicated in her lifetime, a sad testament to our times. But if I've moved you a little closer to the *walls* of the market—the vegeta-ble bins, the whole-wheat breads, the yeast, the whole milk—I count the effort worthwhile.

Neither do I want to preach reform of the food industry. They'll respond only to market pressures—simply because they're not people. They're profit machines. Don't get me wrong: profit is good—for jobs, for investment in new equipment. I don't look for hobgoblins under every bottom line. Yet I think you'll agree that it would be a rare event, not yet encountered in our genera-tion, for a profit machine to offer a food in place of a nonfood with greater profit potential!

To come back to the theme of the Whole Life Diet, listen to Leon Kass of the University of Chicago:

Animals instinctively eat the right foods (when available) and act in such a way as to maintain their naturally given state of health and vigor. Other animals do not overeat, undersleep, knowingly ingest toxic substances, or permit their bodies to fall into disuse through sloth, watching television and riding in automobiles, transacting business or writing articles about health.[4]

So I would say that your duty in the supermarket is to start acting like an animal. Start listening for natural impulses. Stop trusting labels. Stop trusting what doctors say about nutrition. The columnist George F. Will makes a startling point about personal health:

> Today, much illness is willful, in the sense that it results from foolish living habits of people who have a duty to know better. . . . National health insurance might do harm by reinforcing public acceptance of the "no-fault principle" that discounts personal responsibility for health.[5]

That responsibility begins in the supermarket; ironically, it implies hand-to-hand combat with the food merchandisers whom conservatives like Mr. Will seldom question. The enemy in the "combat zones" of the supermarket is at our throats—offering us sugars and hardened fats as if these things were in our best interest. In another age, the high priests were no better, as Mr. Will relates:

> When Shakespeare, Coke, Bacon, and Drake were advancing drama and poetry, jurisprudence, experimental science, navigation and exploration, John Donne, who was doing as much for poetry and preaching, was being treated for fever by doctors who placed a dead pigeon at his feet to draw "vapours" from his brain.[6]

And I must say, at the risk of seeming to be *against* everything rather than *for* something, *stop trusting the government.* The intrusion of the federal agencies of the land into our affairs is no small matter, to be sure—only it affects us more than we think in the *supermarket.* Talk about a combat zone! Listen to this, from a letter to a newspaper from the manufacturer of a sugar-substitute:

> There is something almost obscene in a government subsidizing the tobacco farmer to grow and sell a product that

we know causes cancer in humans and ban the only sugar substitute left. For every pound of saccharin used in this country over 4,000 pounds of sugar are used. Does the F.D.A. contend that one pound of saccharin is more harmful than 4,000 pounds of sugar? Does it matter that heart disease and obesity are almost universally known to be the greatest danger to our health and that the head of the American Heart Association has stated that this ban would cause the death of 25,000 additional heart patients? [7]

I would also ask how many people are killed each year by the RDA labels—sugarcoated with the promise of nutrition.

TWELVE
Making Do in an Imperfect World

We smoke, drink, overeat, rush from place to place, travel at speeds that fool our body's expectation of the cycle of the day. We must frequently eat out. We read conflicting advice. Worst of all, we're told it's all right: processed foods, we are assured, are as good as fresh, and as long as we get the famous "balanced diet" we need no extra effort in our quest for good nutrition.

Listen to what Abram Hoffer says on these two points:

Processed foods provide discord in the metabolic harmony: a missing nutrient is like a fiddle with a broken string. . . . Human metabolism has not adapted to food artifacts recombined into products designed only to please the palate.

. . . The range of variation among individuals is enormous. Some people become violently ill from ingesting foods that are nutritious for others. This truth explodes the myth of the minimum daily requirements (MDR) and recommended daily allowances (RDA) so loved by government agencies. The need for nutrients will vary by many hundred percent.

He sums up:

Thus modern clinical nutrition must be built around two main concepts: the individuality and variability of human beings and the orchestra-like function of nutrients acting in harmony.[1]

Dr. Robert Haskell, a member of the Board of Bariatric Physicians, notes that we spend millions on cancer research, yet conquering cancer would add only two years to the life expectancy of Americans. Conquering obesity, on the other hand, would add seven years to our life expectancy—yet we spend public money to *promote* obesity. Yes—by subsidizing sugar and tobacco.

We live in a contradictory, imperfect world. Up to this point I've said little about this world. I've talked about the ideals—alfalfa tea, cereal bran, crunchy foods, raw vegetables. Yet, like anyone else, I have to travel and eat in unfamiliar places and overcome bad eating habits. I've learned some ways to cope with this world; here are some bits of advice based on my experience.

EATING OUT—AND SURVIVING

Don't Let Restaurants Dictate Your Menu

Restaurants can be safe places to eat if they follow the old-fashioned recipes and avoid hydrogenated oils, deep frying, and charbroiling. Specialty, ethnic menus can add safe calories to a business luncheon or a family celebration. But eating is serious business! It is dangerous to order "blindly" from a menu without knowing how the food is prepared. A simple thing like a hamburger on a bun can be fixed many different ways. Know your shortening, and know your cook!

How easy it is to assume that the chef knows best. To learn otherwise, each of us should work in a restaurant kitchen once in his life!

When You're Hungry, Ask "Is It Safe?"

Whole foods are safest. The baked potato can be carried to the self-service salad bar and loaded with onions, sprouts, and other living things. The poached egg is a delicate item, rich in what the baby chick needed to develop. Raw tomatoes, onions, and other vegetables are nutritious. (We have combined these items into a safe lunch snack: baked potatoes, poached eggs, onions, tomatoes, etc. The safety of this item is the lack of bread —and its possible hydrogenated shortenings.)

When in doubt, substitute a baked potato for the bread.

Soups are safe sources of vegetables and meat because the watery fluids cannot hide unfriendly fat. Grease and lard spoil the flavor quickly. (Grease and lard can be hidden in grilled meats, but not in meats used as a base for soups.) Canned soups are suspect, though, and a trip into the kitchen will clarify what is meant by "home made" on the menu. Remember, keep control of ingredients!

Worry Less about Calories Than about Bad Ingredients

Breads may contain hydrogenated shortening. If they are baked on the premises, you may be able to rule this out. If not, order a baked potato instead.

Ethnic dishes are fine as long as "original ingredients" are used. Most of these dishes originated several generations ago, before the unfriendly fats were developed. It is doubtful that many of our ancestors actually ate rich dishes with the heavy sauces. However, the safety rule to remember is: If my grandmother could have made this dish in her kitchen, then it is safe. I assume that whole foods can't be made too dangerous without modern semisynthetic items.

There is always the danger of too many calories, but a ten-mile run or walk will take care of that. The amount of salt and fat is always more than we need, but such meals can be followed by low-salt and low-fat days of fasting and running. About the only fats to really worry about are the angiotoxic *trans*-fat and cholesterol oxide.

Desserts always have too many calories, too much simple sugar, and often excess fats. However, the caloric balance for the whole day is important in evaluating the wisdom of desserts. Heavy mileage balances heavy desserts!

Hot Grease Ruins Good Food

Avoid menu items that are clearly deep fried. Potatoes, fish, chicken, shrimp, and other whole foods can be covered with sugar, starch, fat, and artificial flavors until there is little food value left. Grease contains toxic lipid oxides because the heat is high enough to burn the fat molecules. Often the menu is vague on the method of cooking; ask the waiter or the manager, or, if you plan on eating there regularly, ask to see the cook!

Keep Alcohol in Scale

I've mentioned some benefits of beer throughout this book. As in anything else, going to extremes is the basic danger.

Beer is food. It comes with the nutrients left over from brewer's yeast and germinated whole grain. Wine is also food—*if* it has been handled correctly. However, there are many semisynthetic "wines" on the market. They have been assembled by food chemists, filtered, colored, and flavored to sell in bulk. If it helps you run, it is probably "real" wine. If it makes it difficult to get out of bed the next day, you have been drinking a poor imitation! Distilled spirits have no nutrients, and excessive intake can damage any organ in the body. When alcohol calories exceed 40 percent of your diet, you are an alcoholic and you are going to get into trouble with your health.

Other People's Smoke Spoils Your Food

The toxic oxides in the tobacco smoke in room air are rapidly absorbed by nonsmokers; because of their healthier lungs they may absorb more nicotine than the smokers. If you absorb a large dose of oxides with your meal, you will cancel out any vitamin E or polyunsaturated EFAs in your meal. Antioxidants in the diet combine with the oxidants from tobacco smoke, leaving you with little nutritional value from the meal. Eat in a no-smoking area if you can; if not, try increasing your intake of vitamin C and vitamin E. I consider secondhand smoke the primary cause of lung cancer in nonsmokers! Therefore, it is really a form of assault; and proper protection should be considered, even if it makes you a bit unpopular!

WHEN YOU TRAVEL, TAKE YOUR
FOOD HABITS WITH YOU

The aerobics generation often finds itself eating in strange places from unfamiliar menus. I joke about getting on a jet plane "with one suitcase of clothing and one suitcase of food." I try to take the things that will be missing from the highly refined, semi-synthetic meals at the strange hotel: bran, yeast, and vitamin C.

Bran: Raw, unprocessed cereal bran can be a lifesaver. For breakfast, I order a cup of hot tea and add a half cup of bran, letting it soak in hot water while I read the morning paper. Then I order a glass of whole milk, adding enough to my bran to give it the consistency of hot cereal. A pinch of sugar is OK. Then I rinse out the cup with milk, drop in the tea bag, ask for more hot water and a lemon wedge and have my tea! At lunch I sprinkle bran on my salad. At supper I let it soak in a glass of beer. By the end of the day I've had my usual fiber intake—with its protective silicon.

Yeast: Read the label on a bottle of brewer's yeast tablets. It has all the water-soluble vitamin B complex plus the essential amino acids. Three tablets will bring each meal up to a high level of nutrition—B vitamins and protein.

Vitamin C: Jet lag, missed sleep, hard racing, and all the stress of spending a few days in a strange place can be met with a few pieces of raw fruit and a couple grams of ascorbic acid. For short trips I try to take enough oranges or apples to last; but on longer stays I have to hunt down a produce source while I'm there.

Beer: Strange cities have strange water; and it takes about a quart of fluid for each hour of running. Your stomach may not be able to adjust to every city's water, but a can of beer is a can of beer. Dehydration can aggravate jet lag and ruin a marathon. A cool can of beer in your hotel room is a handy way to swallow your yeast and bran, and it also meets fluid needs for the kidneys.

PROTECT YOURSELF AGAINST
JET LAG

The stress of readjusting your metabolic clock increases your need for vitamin C. I take a gram for each time zone I cross. But lack of sleep cannot be corrected—without some sleep. Take a brief nap every four hours, long enough to include some good REM time (*rapid eye movement* shows that your brain is at rest and unwinding). Avoid caffeine if you need sleep; it blocks REM and prevents you from taking the protective catnaps.

Drink beer; your body needs more fluids during jet flights because of the faster evaporation at altitude.

Try the *thiamin flush* to keep your mind alert during the time changes: carry yeast tablets at all times.

Try the hot "cup of bran" for breakfast, as outlined above. But save the tea bag for later; the stimulant in the tea can hurt your adjustment to jet lag. The higher bran intake on the trip will balance out the low-fiber content of strange foods in a strange city.

In a sense, the whole modern world is a strange city, and if you want to live a whole life it's up to you to make some serious adjustments. Bon voyage on your journey to age one hundred!

Notes

Chapter One
1. *New England Journal of Medicine* 297:644, 1977.
2. "Stamp Out Food Faddism," *Nutrition Action*, March–April 1975.
3. Abram Hoffer and Morton Walker, *Orthomolecular Nutrition* (New Canaan, Conn.: Keats Publishing, 1978).

Chapter Three
1. *Atherosclerosis* 30:27–43, 1978.
2. *Atherosclerosis* 26:397–403, 1977.
3. *Lancet* 1:454–457, 1977.
4. *British Medical Journal* 1:919, 1978.
5. *Surgery, Gynecology and Obstetrics* 147:49, 1978.
6. *Annals of Internal Medicine* 81:294–301, 1974, and *New England Journal of Medicine* 297:405–409, 1977.
7. *Lancet* 1:538–39, 1977.
8. *Lancet* 2:683, 1978.
9. *Lancet* 2:529, 1978.
10. *Lancet* 2:353, 1978.
11. *British Medical Journal* 1:673, 1978.
12. *New England Journal of Medicine* 298:1005–1007, 1978.
13. *New England Journal of Medicine* 299:419, 1978.

14. *Journal of Clinical Investigation* 48:1313–27, 1969.
15. *Atherosclerosis* 26:29–39, 1977.
16. *Journal of Lipid Research* 8:508–510, 1967.
17. *American Journal of Clinical Nutrition* 32:58–83, 1979.
18. *Surgery* 68:175, 1970.
19. *Atherosclerosis* 21:15–19, 1975.
20. *Journal of the American Geriatrics Society* 17:721–35, 1969.
21. *Lancet* 2:203, 1971.
22. *Journal of the American Oil Chemists' Society* 51:255–59, 1974.
23. *American Heart Journal* 96:569–71, 1978.
24. *Lancet* 2:556, 1977.
25. *New England Journal of Medicine* 297:644, 1977.
26. *Artery* 4:360–84, 1978.
27. *Archives of Pathology and Laboratory Medicine* 100:565–72, 1976.
28. *Atherosclerosis* 28:405–416, 1977.
29. *American Journal of Clinical Nutrition* 31:1041–49, 1978.
30. *New England Journal of Medicine* 296:774–79, 1977.
31. Dr. Carl C. Pfeiffer, *Mental and Elemental Nutrients* (New Canaan, Conn.: Keats Publishing, 1975).

Chapter Four
1. Cited in J. E. Brody, "Chemical Carriers of Cholesterol Put Light on Heart-Attack Puzzle," *New York Times*, 18 January 1977.
2. Dr. Reginald Cherry, 'The Truth about Sugar," *Southwest*, July 1978.

Chapter Five
1. *Lancet* 2:1261, 1978.
2. *Atherosclerosis* 26:397–403, 1977.
3. *Atherosclerosis* 26:397, 1977.
4. *Atherosclerosis* 29:301, 1978.
5. *Atherosclerosis* 19:429–40, 1974.
6. *Lancet* 2:508, 1977.

Chapter Six
1. Karl von Rokitansky, *A Manual of Pathological Anatomy*, vol. 4, trans. G. E. Day (London: Sydenham Society, 1852), pp. 261–72.
2. *Mayo Clinic Proceedings* 53:35, 1978.
3. Rudolf Virchow, *Cellular Pathology as Based upon Physiological and Pathological Histology*, trans. F. Chance (New York: Dover Publications, 1971), pp. 230–54.
4. *Zentralblatt Für Allgermeine Pathologie und Pathologische Anatomie* 24:1–9, 1913.

5. *American Journal of Clinical Nutrition* 21:255, 1968.
6. *Circulation* 59:1–7, 1979.
7. *Lancet* 1:473, 1970.
8. *Lancet* 2:1211, 1978.
9. *Lancet* 2:203–206, 1971.
10. *Journal of the American Geriatrics Society* 17:721, 1969.
11. *British Medical Journal* 2:1307–1314, 1977.
12. *British Medical Journal* 2:1602, 1977.
13. *Proceedings of the Nutrition Society* 17:28, 1958.
14. *New England Journal of Medicine* 289:63–67, 1973.
15. *Circulation Research* 30:675–80, 1972.
16. *American Journal of Clinical Nutrition* 30:664, 1977.
17. *American Journal of Clinical Nutrition* 30:490, 1977.
18. *Clinica Chimica Acta* 1:87, 1964.
19. *American Journal of Clinical Nutrition* 31:1334, 1978.
20. *Atherosclerosis* 26:379–86, 1977.
21. Dr. Johanna Dwyer and Dr. Jean Mayer, "Food for Thought," *San Francisco Examiner*, 20 July 1977.
22. *Nutrition Action*, November–December 1978.
23. *American Journal of Clinical Nutrition* 30:664, 1977 and 30:490, 1977.

Chapter Seven

1. *New England Journal of Medicine* 265:369–73, 1961.
2. *New England Journal of Medicine* 297:543–45, 1977.
3. *American Journal of Clinical Nutrition* 31:2186–97, 1978.
4. *British Medical Journal* 3:254–55, 1970.
5. *Canadian Medical Association Journal* 107:503–508, 1972.
6. *Proceedings of the National Academy of Sciences of the United States of America* 70:969–72, 1973.
7. *Lancet* 2:544–46, 1974.
8. *Proceedings of the National Academy of Sciences of the United States of America* 70:1461–63, 1973.
9. *Oncology* 27:181–92, 1973.
10. *Journal of Urology* 103:155–59, 1970.
11. *Lancet* 2:607, 1977.
12. *Chemico-Biological Interactions* 9:285–315, 1974.
13. *Proceedings of the National Academy of Sciences of the United States of America* 73:3685–89, 1976.
14. *Nature* 225:744–45, 1970.
15. *Lancet* 1:247, 1976.
16. *Lancet* 1:798, 1972.
17. *Annals of Internal Medicine* 90:85–91, 1979.
18. *Annals of Internal Medicine* 84:385–88, 1976.

19. *American Journal of Clinical Nutrition* 31:1397–99, 1978.
20. *Lancet* 1:491, 1972.
21. *Nature* 238:277, 1972.
22. *Surgery, Gynecology and Obstetrics* 147:49–55, 1978.
23. *New England Journal of Medicine* 299:317–23, 1978.
24. *New England Journal of Medicine* 299:1319, 1978.
25. *American Journal of Clinical Nutrition* 31:253–58, 1978.
26. *American Journal of Clinical Nutrition* 28:1381–86, 1975.
27. *Nutrition Reports International* 11:473, 1975.
28. *Research Communications in Chemical Pathology and Pharmacology* 7:783, 1974.
29. *Archives of Environmental Health* 30:234, 1975.
30. *Journal of Clinical Investigation* 57:732, 1976.
31. *Proceedings of the Society for Experimental Biology and Medicine* 149:275, 1975.
32. *British Journal of Nutrition* 26:89, 1971.
33. *Lancet* 1:1155–57, 1973.
34. *American Journal of Clinical Nutrition* 27:1179, 1974.
35. *American Journal of Clinical Nutrition* 29:569–78, 1976.

Chapter Nine
1. *Proceedings of the Royal Society of Medicine* 57:23, 1964.
2. *Atherosclerosis* 26:379–86, 1977.
3. *Atherosclerosis* 21:15, 1975.
4. *Advances in Enzymology and Related Areas of Molecular Biology* 11:377, 1951.
5. *Annals of Internal Medicine* 90:85–91, 1979.
6. *Lancet* 1:72–75, 1979.
7. *New England Journal of Medicine* 297:644–50, 1977.
8. O. Appenzeller and R. Atkinson, eds., *Health Aspects of Endurance Training*, Medicine and Sport Series, vol. 12 (Basel, Switzerland: S. Karger Publishers, 1978), pp. 88–104.
9. *American Journal of Clinical Nutrition* 27:1182, 1974.

Chapter Ten
1. *Lancet* 2:204, 1978.
2. *New York Times*, 28 January 1979.
3. *Lancet* 2:671–74, 1972.
4. *Lancet* 2:1261, 1978.

Chapter Eleven
1. Cited in Dr. Harold Rosenberg with A. N. Feldzamen, Ph.D., *The Book of Vitamin Therapy* (New York: Berkley, Windhover, 1975), p. 28.

2. Cited in Dr. Harold Rosenberg with A. N. Feldzamen, Ph.D, *The Book of Vitamin Therapy* (New York: Berkley, Windhover, 1975), p. 34.
3. *Journal of the American Geriatrics Society* 17:721, 1969.
4. "A Right to Health," *Newsweek*, 17 August 1978.
5. "A Right to Health," *Newsweek*, 17 August 1978.
6. "A Right to Health," *Newsweek*, 17 August 1978.
7. Benjamin J. Eisenstadt, *New York Times*, 19 April 1977.

Chapter Twelve
1. Abram Hoffer and Morton Walker, *Orthomolecular Nutrition* (New Canaan, Conn.: Keats Publishing, 1978).